Life-threate

Allerg
Reactions

Understanding

& Coping with

Anaphylaxis

C000076151

By the same authors

Asthma: The complete guide for sufferers and carers

Life-threatening Allergic Reactions

Understanding

& Coping with

Anaphylaxis

Dr DERYK WILLIAMS,
ANNA WILLIAMS
AND LAURA CROKER

PIATKUS

This book is dedicated to Weymouth Grammar School, with thanks

© 1997 Dr Deryk Williams, Anna Williams and Laura Croker

First published in 1997 by
Judy Piatkus (Publishers) Ltd
5 Windmill Street, London W1P 1HF

The moral right of the authors has been asserted

A catalogue record for this book
is available from the British Library

ISBN 0-7499-1700-8 pbk

Edited by Kelly Davis
Designed by Sue Ryall
Artworks by Jane Upton and One-Eleven Line Art

Set in Plantin by Action Typesetting, Gloucester
Printed and bound in Great Britain by
Biddles Ltd, Guildford & King's Lynn

CONTENTS

ACKNOWLEDGEMENTS

We would like to thank the following people and organisations for the help they have given us: The Anaphylaxis Campaign, Suzanne Allan, Juliet Burt, Glynis Boddy, British Allergy Foundation, David Chapman, Dr George Chew, Teresa Chris, Hazel Gowland, Annabelle Hancock, Susan Hill, Anne Lawrance, Christine Livingston, Barbara Middleton, Alison Randall, Caroline Rawlinson, David Reading, Anita Roberts, David Steinhoff, Jane Upton, Professor David Warrell and Mandy Vanstone.

FOREWORD

This is an important book for sufferers from anaphylaxis (the life-threatening allergic reaction to many substances), for those with and among whom they live and work, and for the medical profession. Precisely what any of us are so severely allergic to is of importance to us, because we need to avoid it, and to be helped to do so by others. But it is the reaction itself, its severity and swiftness, that needs to be even more widely and clearly recognised and correctly treated. That the right, life-saving treatment is available and relatively simple is one of the principle messages of this book.

Anaphylaxis kills. I know. In the summer of 1995, I almost died of it, after a wasp sting. I knew that I was severely allergic to the stings and had undergone a long course of desenitisation treatment to try and decrease my sensitivity. The treatment failed; it sometimes does. Since then I have always carried adrenaline – even those whose desensitisation has apparently been successful are recommended never to be without it. I had some there, in my bedroom, on the night I was stung. Nevertheless, I nearly lost my life, partly because of a misplaced sense of caution about administering what I had regarded as an extremely dangerous drug, and also because of a common and particularly worrying feature of this condition – denial. Perhaps it wasn't really a wasp – perhaps it won't really be serious this time ... perhaps I ought not to make a huge fuss. I'll just wait and see... I did not use my adrenaline at once, I rang my GP who, thank God, was at home nearby. When he arrived less than ten minutes later, my blood pressure was dropping so low, so quickly, that he was obliged to give me a mega-dose of adrenaline intravenously (potentially a far more dangerous procedure than my having self-administered smaller doses intra-muscularly). He was obliged to do a lot of other dramatic things too, but I still almost died, notably of pulmonary oedema. My lungs filled with fluid and blood, I spent a terrifying twenty-minute ambulance journey, close to death, eleven days in hospital, and several weeks in physical and, even more important, psychological convalescence.

This book may save someone else, perhaps many other people, from that experience. There is still widespread confusion, ignorance and misinformation on the subject of life-threatening allergic reactions, partly because the word 'allergy' has been hi-jacked by some dubious practitioners of, to say the least, unproven theories. I was recently told earnestly by a woman that she had taken her son to an alternative clinic and, via hair-testing, discovered that he was allergic to a wide range of foods and substances, from fresh orange juice and cheese to synthetic fabrics and that these were causing his dyslexia and other learning difficulties. It has become fashionable to suffer from allergies. It is perhaps yet more shocking that even some doctors mistreat, or under-treat severe allergic reactions. Last year, a woman was reported to have died of a bee sting, in spite of having swallowed an antihistamine tablet which she carried for such emergencies. Her doctor had told her – because, I am sure, he believed it – that antihistamine by mouth would give her adequate protection in the event of a sting. How many others in the medical profession still believe that?

This book does not pull punches. It clarifies the condition, it is straightforward and gets its message across urgently. That message is simple. Anaphylaxis kills, perhaps more often than has previously been supposed. It can masquerade as an asthma attack (to which it may be medically related), a heart attack and even a panic attack. Some of their symptoms are identical. But it is also worth mentionng that, as with many other medical conditions, not every case of anaphylaxis presents in the same, classical way. Most sufferers have immediate swelling of the throat and breathing difficulties. I do not. My blood pressure simply drops, very fast. I go sheetwhite, have a dreadful sense of restlessness, panic and foreboding. My pulse races, I breathe easily, but very fast.

So how can others recognise anaphylaxis? One of the essential messages contained in these pages, which all sufferers must take on board, is that often they cannot. The first person who knows what is happening and why, and what to do about it, is the one having the life-threatening reaction. We know what has triggered it – with luck; we should carry our life-saving adrenaline, use it at once, and use it repeatedly; we should call for help and if possible explain exactly how that help needs to be given.

I have to plan my daily life, for the rest of my life, around the avoidance of wasps – and not, as is commonly supposed only in the summer; wasps can crawl out of cracks or be lurking in curtain folds inside the house during the coldest winter months too. I wear a MedicAlert necklet and disc at all times, I carry adrenaline on my person, have it in every room of the house and in my handbag, together with a back-up pack of antihistamine and steroids. If I am likely to be at the slightest risk in any situation, I tell those around me of my condition and what they should do to help me if I am stung – that can be done briefly and simply, without making a fuss. In short, like all sufferers from possible anaphylaxis, I am primarily responsible for myself and my condition. In that sense, I am no different to a sufferer from diabetes or epilepsy.

Apart from the reaction itself, the worst thing we have to fear is *fear*. I had a post-traumatic stress condition for months after my near-death anaphylaxis. I was terrified to go out, I had nightmares, I saw a wasp in every midge and fly. I got a small splinter in my hand and knew, *saw* that it was a splinter – but my body went into a huge panic reaction, with breathlessness, pallor, racing heart, faintness, sense of doom, all the symptoms of a real attack. To walk about the world with this time-bomb ticking away is very likely to cause panic at the slightest provocation. That psychological condition has to be dealt with too.

Is there any hope? Has this book any help to offer us? Goodness, yes. Quite apart from the research being done on several fronts into life-threatening allergic reactions and very likely to prove fruitful in one way or another in the long term, the most important message is that we are extremely lucky people. For the most part, we know what triggers our reaction, and our life-saving emergency treatment is freely available to us in an easily and speedily administered form. We can save our own lives. You can't say that about most life-threatening medical conditions. We can also plan to avoid the substances to which we are allergic, coolly and intelligently. We can learn both to minimise risk and yet always bear it in mind, to fear what may kill us, without crippling ourselves with fear. A tall order, a challenge – yes. And possible? Yes, certainly.

This book contains a full and clear introduction to life-threatening allergic reactions for everyone. For myself, and other sufferers, its message is straightforward. Potentially, our condition could not be more serious and, for the foreseeable future at least, we have to live with it. We do not have to die from it.

Susan Hill
Gloucestershire, 1996

1

THE FACTS ABOUT ANAPHYLAXIS

MAN DIES FROM WASP STING

WOMAN KILLED BY WALNUT BUTTER

TEST TO FIGHT PEANUT DEATHS

Newspaper headlines such as these are becoming increasingly common. They all refer to a condition known as anaphylaxis which causes severe, uncontrolled allergic reactions. It is a condition that can kill.

You may worry about shocking headlines like these, or perhaps you dismiss them as unnecessarily sensational. After all, do we really need more scare stories? Unfortunately, in this case we do, because allergies can kill, and people do die. Yet many people and even some doctors are still unaware or misinformed about anaphylaxis.

Having an anaphylactic attack is a terrifying experience that can have a huge impact on your life. These attacks are usually triggered by mundane, everyday events, like being stung by a wasp, eating peanuts or wearing rubber gloves. Being anaphylactic can mean being on guard for the rest of your life.

If you have had a bad reaction to a wasp sting you may be too scared to venture out of doors during the summer.

Peanuts are a very common hidden ingredient in many foods: people who are highly allergic to peanuts sometimes compare going out for a meal to playing a game of Russian roulette. Someone who knows they are anaphylactic can feel as if they are a human time bomb, liable to detonate at any moment.

However, being anaphylactic need not mean living in a state of fear. Sensible professional advice and up-to-date information can take the shock out of the headlines and make anaphylaxis manageable. In this book we will show you how to reduce the chances of anaphylaxis developing in the first place, and how to be in control of established anaphylaxis so as to minimise its impact on your life.

BARBARA'S STORY

Barbara's anaphylactic attack was so dramatic that it was reconstructed on British television to try and inform people about the dangers of anaphylaxis:

'I had just put on a brand new pair of rubber gloves, and in minutes my hands began to itch. I had never felt anything like it before. I had to rip off the gloves, and the itching was so intense that I was tearing the skin as I scratched it. I tried to wash my hands, but they swelled as if they were filling up with water. My skin went transparent and I could see lumps underneath. My nose streamed, my eyes pricked and my eyelids swelled all round my eyeballs which had become like thick jelly.'

Barbara suffers from hayfever, asthma and eczema, and had previously had mild reactions to nuts. These were enough to make her realise that this reaction was very serious. She tried to take antihistamines, but lumps were forming in her mouth. On the advice of her doctor, her son took her to hospital. On arrival, Barbara was unable to see or speak, and she felt as if her hands and face were going to burst.

She was taken straight into the casualty department where she was given adrenaline, nebulised salbutamol, hydrocortisone and piriton and put on a heart monitor (see Chapter 5 on treatments).

After 15 minutes she felt that the attack was beginning to subside. She remained on a heart monitor for two days, and after five days the swelling in her face and hands began to go down.

Barbara was fearful of leaving hospital, but has since learned to cope with her fear. She always carries adrenaline, and now wears a MedicAlert bracelet (see p. 67) for quick emergency response. Latex is to be avoided at all costs, as well as other triggers like cats, dogs and even some kinds of soap.

Barbara's work as a school secretary enables her to help spread awareness about the seriousness of anaphylaxis and how to deal with it. 'The more people know about this condition,' she says, 'the more likely they are to act quickly and prevent a disaster.'

Anaphylaxis Past and Present

Despite today's screaming headlines, anaphylaxis is nothing new. Food has been known to cause harmful reactions in susceptible individuals for 2000 years. Both Hippocrates, the Greek physician and 'Father of Medicine', and Galen, physician, philosopher and for centuries the supreme medical authority, were aware of and recorded an intolerance of milk. The Roman poet Lucretius, who died in 55BC, wrote these wise words in *De Rerum Natura*: 'Ut quod ali cibus est aliis fuat acre venemum,' or as we would say, 'One man's meat is another man's poison.'

We now know that anaphylactic attacks are a lot more common than was once thought. Throughout North America, Europe and Japan, about 12,000 people suffer an anaphylactic attack each year. Around 360 people, or possibly more, will die from one of these. The most common causes are insect stings and food allergies. In North America, Europe and Japan, it is estimated that a further seven million people who have a family history of allergies may develop anaphylactic reactions.

Recent scientific evidence suggests that the number of people currently identified as having died of an anaphylactic attack may very well be hugely underestimated. As we will see, people who suffer from asthma are at a higher risk of developing anaphylaxis. It is now thought that as many as 15 per cent of sudden deaths attributed to asthma are in fact caused by anaphylactic attacks. In the UK alone this would increase the number of deaths that can be attributed each year to anaphylaxis by around 300.

Deaths from anaphylaxis occur largely because of ignorance. Nearly all anaphylaxis deaths could be prevented. This book will help you to deal confidently and effectively with a life-threatening allergic reaction – and so save a life.

What Can We Do?

There are three key points to remember in order to deal successfully with anaphylaxis: Recognition, Avoidance and Treatment – RAT.

First, you must be able to RECOGNISE an anaphylactic attack. Often, full-blown anaphylaxis is preceded by a milder allergic-type reaction on a previous occasion. You, or your doctor, may not recognise the significance of this early reaction, and you could therefore be left in a vulnerable situation. A full-blown anaphylactic attack may be confused with other medical emergencies, such as severe asthma or a heart attack. If the anaphylactic reaction is not recognised, life-saving treatment cannot be administered. Chapter 4 explains how to recognise anaphylaxis.

Most people who have had an anaphylactic attack know what caused it. If the cause is not apparent, it is essential to try and find out what it is. When you know what caused your anaphylaxis, you must then AVOID this factor. For example, if you are allergic to peanuts you must have good knowledge of food labelling and the content of various foods. In Chapter 3, we investigate this in detail.

The main TREATMENT for anaphylaxis is an injection of adrenaline. (In many other countries, adrenaline is known as epinephrine.) In anaphylaxis, adrenaline is life-saving. However, it must be given at the beginning of an anaphylactic attack. If you have experienced anaphylaxis before, it is crucial that you carry an adequate supply of adrenaline on you at *all* times. Chapter 5 gives detailed information about the medication used to treat anaphylaxis.

In this book we will show you how to **recognise** anaphylaxis, how to identify and **avoid** the factors that provoke anaphylaxis, and, should anaphylaxis occur, how to **treat** it quickly and effectively.

ALICIA'S STORY

Two-year-old Alicia was diagnosed as having peanut allergy at the age of 13 months. She attends the crèche at the hospital where her mother works as a midwife. The manager and staff of the crèche have worked closely with Alicia's mother and with healthcare professionals to develop a strategy for minimising risks to Alicia.

One day the crèche manager telephoned Alicia's mother to say that she was having a reaction: the first one since being diagnosed as peanut allergic. Her mother arrived within minutes and gave the dose of adrenaline to her screaming daughter. By this time her daughter's face was red and swollen, and her eyes were almost closed. If Alicia's mother had not been immediately available one of the staff would have given the adrenaline. Alicia was taken to the accident and emergency department, and spent the afternoon on a ward, until she was fully recovered.

So, what went wrong? The hospital chef had cooked the lunchtime chips in the fryer previously used to fry nut cutlets. Alicia ate only half a chip, but this was enough to provoke an anaphylactic reaction.

2

WHAT IS ANAPHYLAXIS?

The term anaphylaxis is derived from the Greek words *ana*, meaning 'excessive', and *phylaxis*, meaning 'protection'. It may seem bizarre but an anaphylactic reaction actually begins as a protective mechanism. If this mechanism is not turned off it gets out of control and can end up by damaging us.

The Inflammatory Response

Anaphylaxis begins with an entirely normal bodily reaction, *the inflammatory response* (see diagram on p. 9). Our bodies use this response to protect us from hostile factors in the environment, such as infections or noxious chemicals. The problem with anaphylaxis is that the inflammatory response goes out of control and for some reason the body cannot switch it off. To understand how this has come about, we need to look at how the body uses the inflammatory response to protect itself from hostile factors in the environment.

We are all familiar with the inflammatory response. For example, if you were to spill hot water on your arm, there would be redness and swelling. The redness is caused by the blood vessels becoming wider and increasing the blood flow;

the swelling is caused by the blood vessels becoming leaky.

For an inflammatory response to occur, your body needs white blood cells, antibodies and powerful chemicals called *inflammatory mediators*. These circulate in the bloodstream, and pass through blood vessel walls and between cells.

The inflammatory response starts when a factor is identified as being hostile and antibodies attach themselves to it. The antibodies cause the white blood cells to discharge inflammatory mediators, and the inflammatory mediators cause the blood vessels surrounding the hostile factor to become wider and to become leaky. This increases the supply of blood in order to rush fresh supplies of white blood cells, antibodies and inflammatory mediators into the area. The white blood cells, antibodies and inflammatory mediators then interact to break down and remove the hostile factor and so combat the threat to your body.

An allergic reaction occurs when your body mounts an inflammatory response against a harmless factor. Since the factor is harmless, this is called an *inappropriate* inflammatory response. The factor that causes such a response is called an *allergen*. Pollen is a common example of an allergen. People who suffer from hayfever are allergic to pollen. When they breathe in, there is an inappropriate inflammatory reaction in the lining of the nose. The leaky blood vessels cause the nose to drip, and the lining of the nose becomes red and inflamed.

Inflammation and Anaphylaxis

In an anaphylactic attack an allergic reaction escalates out of control, resulting in *systemic inflammation* (inflammation throughout your body). This means that your blood vessels widen and become leaky, causing different effects in different parts of your body. On your skin big blisters called weals may appear. In your mouth your tongue may swell up. Inflammation in your intestines may cause you to have

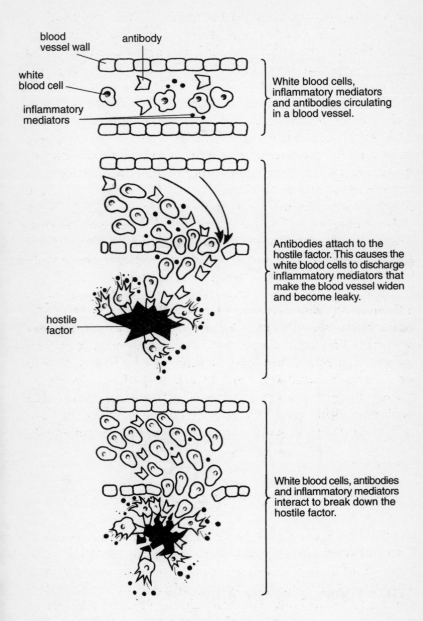

The inflammatory response

diarrhoea or you may vomit. Your hands may appear to fill up with water, as if you were wearing transparent gloves.

The two areas where the most dangerous effects of systemic inflammation occur are in your airways and in your circulatory system.

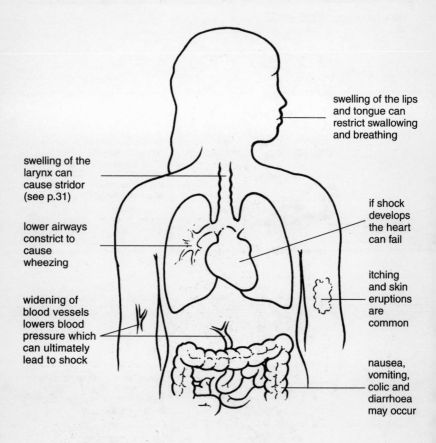

swelling of the lips and tongue can restrict swallowing and breathing

swelling of the larynx can cause stridor (see p.31)

lower airways constrict to cause wheezing

widening of blood vessels lowers blood pressure which can ultimately lead to shock

if shock develops the heart can fail

itching and skin eruptions are common

nausea, vomiting, colic and diarrhoea may occur

The effects of anaphylaxis on different parts of the body

WHAT HAPPENS IN THE AIRWAYS?

Your airways are constructed like an upside-down tree. The large upper airways are the windpipe (*trachea*), and the voice box (*larynx*). The lower airways (*bronchi*) enter your lungs, and repeatedly branch into tiny airways called *bronchioles*. These end in collections of air-filled sacs (*alveoli*) which look like bunches of grapes. It is in the alveoli that oxygen from the air you breathe passes into your bloodstream, so that it can be carried to every cell in your body.

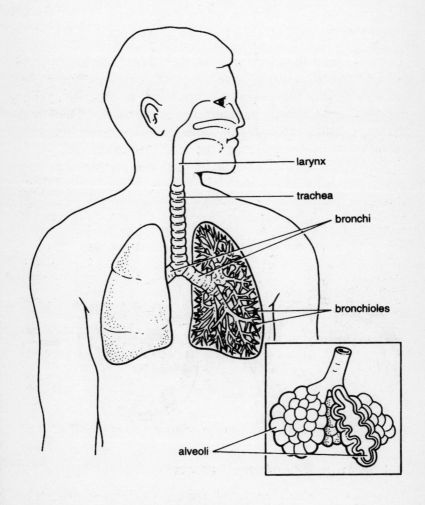

larynx

trachea

bronchi

bronchioles

alveoli

Inside the lungs

The problem is that the outside of all but the smallest airways is fairly rigid. When inflammation occurs in the lining of the airway, the lining becomes swollen but can only expand into the central hollow or *lumen* (see below). The airways gets so narrow that very little air can get through. This makes breathing extremely difficult, and ultimately impossible, resulting in respiratory arrest and death.

What Happens in the Circulatory System?

The heart and blood vessels together form your circulatory system. The heart is really a very sophisticated pump. Its function is to pump blood around your body, in order to supply every cell in your body with oxygen and nutrients. The blood vessels passing through the lungs collect oxygen, and the blood vessels passing through the gut collect nutrients.

When there is an anaphylactic reaction, the blood vessels

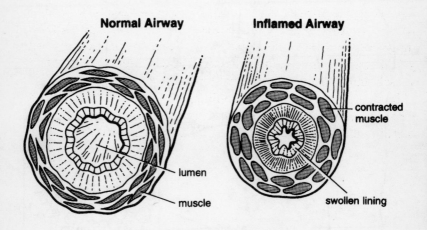

The inside of a normal and an inflamed airway

widen and become leaky, and there is less and less blood available for your heart to pump. Ultimately, if there is insufficient blood being pumped by your heart to meet the needs of your body, you go into a state of *shock*.

Shock is a very serious medical condition. In anaphylaxis, shock occurs because the inflammation causes a critically low blood supply to important organs such as the lungs, kidneys, liver, gut, and perhaps most importantly the brain. If shock is not successfully treated, all these vital organs become starved of oxygen and nutrients, resulting in multi-organ failure and death.

There is an important distinction to be drawn here between medical shock and other uses of the word, such as being 'shocked' by a sudden noise. The former is very serious, the latter is not.

To recap, anaphylaxis is a severe allergic reaction, which results in inflammation throughout the body. Anaphylaxis is dangerous because inflammation in the airways may prevent you from breathing, and leaking and widening of blood vessels may lead to circulatory collapse.

In order to prevent anaphylaxis, we need to understand what causes it. The next chapter describes the different factors which trigger this excessive allergic reaction.

3

WHAT CAUSES ANAPHYLAXIS?

Anaphylaxis is caused by a substance or factor to which the anaphylactic person is highly allergic. The most common causes of anaphylaxis are foodstuffs, especially nuts. There are also thousands of people whose anaphylaxis is caused by insect stings, latex, some drugs, exercise, stress or a combination of these. There are some people whose anaphylaxis seems to have no particular cause, and others whose anaphylaxis is caused by rare or unusual factors.

Nuts and Seeds

PEANUTS

The average American eats roughly 11lb (5kg) of peanut products each year – about half of this as peanut butter and the rest in sweets, baked foods and nuts. Although the rest of us may not consume quite so many peanuts, they are enormously popular all over the world.

The peanut is actually a kind of bean from the leguminous plant *arachis hypogaea*, which comes from tropical America. It is cultivated for its edible seeds, which are forced underground to ripen. A few people who are allergic to peanuts

14

may also develop allergies to other legumes such as soya, peas and beans.

In recent years the peanut has been branded a killer. 'CHILDREN IN PERIL FROM PEANUTS' scream the headlines, chilling those for whom anaphylaxis is a fact of life. The real killer, of course, is our own ignorance, and our unpreparedness to cope with the dangers peanuts *might* present, especially when their presence is hidden.

SARAH'S STORY

Sarah had suffered from asthma since the age of three. She had been in hospital several times with bad attacks of asthma. These attacks usually happened after she had had a bad cold which then went to her chest. She also suffered from eczema, and was moderately allergic to various foods including dairy products, cucumber and peanuts. Sarah was aware of which foods triggered her allergic reactions, and was careful to avoid them.

In 1993, when she was 17 years old, Sarah came back from a shopping trip feeling unwell. She was wheezing, and her mouth felt strange. She said this was different from a normal asthma attack. As her breathing deteriorated, her stepmother called the doctor, who advised taking Sarah to the surgery immediately. But it was too late. Sarah collapsed and died within minutes.

The mystery of her death was explained when a till receipt was found in her handbag, showing that she had eaten a slice of lemon meringue pie in a chain store restaurant. When the ingredients of the pie were examined, it was found to have been garnished with a sprinkling of crushed peanuts. Sarah had died of anaphylactic shock caused by eating crushed peanuts.

The increase in peanut-induced anaphylaxis may be partly due to the early age at which children are being given peanuts. The mother who smears a crust of bread with smooth peanut butter and then presents it to her baby as a first finger food may unwittingly be *sensitising* her child to peanuts, thus setting up the mechanism that could lead to a life-threatening anaphylactic attack.

A recent study at the Isle of Wight Allergy Research Unit discovered that one in 75 children had been sensitised to peanuts by the age of four (although this does not mean that all those children will be at risk from severe anaphylaxis). In Southampton, a major new peanut research project has found that more children are becoming sensitised to peanuts at an early age, and has suggested that babies can even be sensitised to peanuts and other allergens through breast milk.

SENSITISING

People who have allergies are likely to have an *atopic tendency*. This means that their genes give them a tendency to develop allergies. The same genes will also make them likely to suffer from hayfever, asthma and eczema. The atopic tendency runs in families, which is why you may find that, if you are anaphylactic, your close relatives may well be asthmatics, or hayfever or eczema sufferers. Having an atopic tendency does not necessarily mean that you will develop any of the above conditions, but it is likely.

In anaphylaxis, when you first encounter the factor that causes your allergic reaction there may be no visible reaction to it. However, from then on, you have been *sensitised* to that factor: your immune system has noted it, mistakenly identified it as a hostile factor and alerted your body to react strongly whenever it is encountered (see Chapter 2).

A major peanut product is *peanut oil*, which is extracted from pressed peanuts. This oil is used in cooking, in the manufacture of soaps and in pharmaceutical products. Some of the creams which breastfeeding mothers use to soothe cracked nipples contain peanut oil under a different name – arachis oil. This is inevitably ingested by babies along with their milk. Arachis oil is also present in some of the creams used to soothe nappy rash and could then be absorbed through cracked skin.

It's important to be aware of other names, or 'aliases', for peanuts and peanut oil. Peanuts are also known as ground nuts, monkey nuts, goobers, and goober peas. And peanut oil is also known as arachis oil, ground nut oil and may be a constituent of vegetable oil. Recently it has been suggested that refined peanut oil may not be allergenic. Research, however, is ongoing.

FOODSTUFFS AND PREPARATIONS WHICH MAY CONTAIN PEANUTS OR PEANUT OIL

Peanuts:
peanut butter, chocolate-covered nuts, chocolate bars, confectionery, bread, biscuits, cakes, pastries, ice cream desserts, mixed nuts, trail mix, salted peanuts, breakfast cereals, almond icing, Chinese food, Thai food, Indonesian food, satay sauce, curries, chilli, salads, gravy, spaghetti sauce, vegeburgers, vegetarian foods, salad dressings and garnishes for many foods.

Peanut oil:
cooking oils, jelly, ice cream cones and wafers, soup, tinned sardines, margarine, cooking fats, some baby milk powders, breast cream, baby creams, ear drops, dressings, antibiotic creams, other creams used in dentistry, lipsticks, massage oils.

OTHER NUTS

Anaphylaxis can also be caused by 'real' nuts (sometimes called 'tree nuts'), such as brazils, almonds, walnuts, hazels or cashews. Nuts are widely used in food production, and are not necessarily apparent in either the food's taste or its appearance. In 1995 a woman collapsed and died after eating walnut butter at a Manchester Christmas party. She knew she was allergic to nuts, but did not realise they were an ingredient of her meal.

Reactions to nuts are not only caused by eating them. Aromatherapy, a popular area of complementary healthcare, uses mixtures of fragrant and often potent massage oils to try to relieve particular ailments in individuals. Almond oil is a common ingredient of aromatherapy oils, and this has been known to cause an attack in an anaphylactic patient who did not realise that nut oil was being rubbed all over her body.

Whilst it is apparent from these examples that we need to be vigilant about checking for the presence of peanuts and tree nuts, it is important to balance this with the knowledge that adrenaline, the antidote to anaphylaxis, is accessible, portable and effective (see Chapter 5). Anyone who has experienced a serious anaphylactic attack is greatly reassured by knowing what their medical problem is, and that they can always carry the medication to counteract this problem with them.

RACHEL'S STORY

One day last year Rachel was eating her sandwiches at school with her friends. One friend offered a sandwich to another and Rachel obligingly took it and handed it across. Then she absent-mindedly licked her fingers. The sandwich contained peanut butter and Rachel suffered a serious allergic reaction. But that week Rachel's teachers had received training in the use of the adrenaline injection – and the headmaster administered the adrenaline to Rachel. His quick action probably saved her life.

SESAME SEEDS

Sesame (*Sesamum indicum*) has been grown since ancient times, and is cultivated in Africa, Eastern Europe, India, China and Central America. Sesame is high in protein, and the seeds, which are enclosed in the fruit, are ground and used in *tahini* and other traditional dishes. Sesame oil is extracted from sesame seeds, usually by the traditional process of heating, pressing and extracting. Oil can also be obtained by 'cold pressing'. Cold-pressed oil is thought to be more likely to cause problems for people with anaphylaxis, as high temperatures may destroy the allergens in the seed.

A number of people have experienced extreme allergic reactions to sesame seeds. With the move towards healthier eating, sesame seeds appear regularly in vegetarian food, often as a hidden ingredient in sauces, pastes and mixed spices. They are also more likely to appear in children's food, as well as being scattered on top of the ubiquitous burger bun. Sesame even turns up on the ingredients lists of some 'healthy' sparkling drinks. Sesame oil is also used widely in Chinese and Greek cooking, and can be found in skin creams.

Other Foodstuffs

Various foods are known to have caused mild or severe anaphylactic attacks. These include fish, shellfish, fruit, vegetables and cereals. It is important to be aware that, because it is an allergic reaction, anaphylaxis can be triggered by almost anything. Anyone looking for the cause of an attack should not limit themselves to the known triggers, but investigate all possibilities.

This is especially difficult with processed foods, because it is sometimes difficult to discover exactly what is in them. In Chapter 6 we will examine food labelling, and look at how the food industry is dealing with the awareness that food containing even the merest trace of an allergen has the potential to kill.

DAIRY PRODUCTS

As we have seen, allergies to milk are nothing new: there are records of this occurring in the Roman times. A number of studies have shown that between 2 and 3 per cent of young infants may be allergic to cow's milk protein. Formula milk and soya milk can both cause allergic reactions in babies. The good news is that approximately 75 per cent of children who were allergic to cow's milk in infancy can tolerate milk by the age of four or five.

EGGS

Eggs are the most common food allergen affecting babies between the ages of six and nine months. Again, many children grow out of this allergy. The main egg allergen is found in the egg white. The measles, mumps and rubella vaccine (MMR) is grown in cultures made from chicken embryos. It is possible that a child who is allergic to eggs will also react to this vaccine. Generally the MMR can still be given, but under careful medical supervision.

Insect Stings

The venom in some insect stings contains a potent, complex mixture of allergens including enzymes, histamines and other proteins. Because the mixture is so complex, there is no single antidote to insect sting venom.

Between 15 and 25 per cent of the population will have an allergic reaction to insect sting venom, although this does not mean that they are all at risk from a life-threatening allergic reaction. The risk of death from insect sting anaphylaxis is greater in adults over 40 years of age. In Britain the ratio of such deaths between men and women is about equal. In America between 50 and 150 people die annually from insect sting anaphylaxis.

Just as there are probably more anaphylaxis deaths generally than those officially recorded, it is likely that there are more deaths from insect sting anaphylaxis than those recorded. A study in 1995 showed that in seven out of 27 unexplained sudden deaths there were antibodies to venom present in the body, suggesting that the person had recently been stung.

The insect family whose members inflict stings which can result in serious allergic reactions is called *Hymenoptera*. There are three major problem groups from this family: *apids, vespids* and *formicids*.

BEES

Apids include honey bees and bumble bees. Honey bees may sting to defend their colony, and so beekeepers are greatly at risk of becoming sensitised to their venom. Bumble bees are seldom aggressive.

WASPS AND HORNETS

Vespids include wasps, hornets and paper wasps. Wasps are highly aggressive, especially as the end of summer approaches and their sources of food become scarce. They scavenge in highly populated areas such as beaches, parks, gardens and around rubbish bins. Wasps are the most common cause of anaphylaxis from insect stings, and cause twice as many deaths as bee stings. The stings which are most dangerous are those to the head or neck, leading quickly to obstruction of the airways.

The danger caused by wasp venom is ever-present. Often people are stung by wasps in the house, where they had thought they would be safe. One woman suffered a severe anaphylactic attack after brushing against the sting of a dead wasp which had fallen into her bed, and a man died after treading on a wasp in his garden. Anita's story shows just how dangerous, and frightening, wasps can be.

ANITA'S STORY

Anita lives amidst glorious English countryside, near fields of linseed and bright yellow rape. When the pollen count is high she suffers from dry, gritty eyes and blocked sinuses. Now aged 52, Anita had never been stung by a wasp until seven years ago.

Unbeknown to Anita, there was a wasps' nest in the eaves above her bedroom. Initially, she was stung on her side, and a huge red lump appeared. Then 10 days later, she was stung twice in one night, just below her knee. Her leg ballooned and she felt as if an electric shock were passing through her entire body. Even the pressure of clothes was too much to bear. When she visited her doctor Anita was told that the sting 'must have hit a nerve', and was given antibiotics. Incredibly, 10 days later, she was stung again.

This time Anita encountered the big reaction. Her skin became bright red and covered in welts; she began to swell up. As the inside of her mouth and throat began to tighten and constrict, she had difficulty breathing. She felt frightened, doomed; she was fading in and out of consciousness. Her husband called the doctor – thankfully not the one she had seen before – and Anita was given adrenaline. The attack subsided and after five days she began to feel better.

Nowadays, Anita controls the likelihood of having another anaphylactic attack by always carrying an injection of adrenaline, as well as antihistamines. She keeps

---

all the windows in her house closed, avoids the beach and swimming pools and hardly ever drives on her own.

But she is still worried. 'I don't like being on my own any more,' she says. 'I am terrified of having another attack. I know that I am lucky in that my attack was dealt with in time, and yet at times, I am like a neurotic wreck. I hate going shopping, I am frightened of the wasps that hover around rubbish bins. I would like to visit old friends in California, but I am worried about how I would cope with the wasps there. There is never a day goes by when I haven't got eyes like a hawk's, looking for the wasps. The anxiety is always there. I know it sounds dramatic, but I tend to think that each wasp I see is the one that is looking out for me ...'

Hornets are very large brown wasps which are found less frequently and rarely attack people. They are most common around old woodlands in Southern England. Paper wasps tend to live in the warmer areas of Southern Europe.

FIRE ANTS AND HARVESTER ANTS

Formicids include fire ants and harvester ants. They tend to live in America, where sensitisation to their stings is a major cause of anaphylactic attacks.

Although not a member of the *Hymenoptera* family, another native of America with a sting that can cause anaphylaxis is the *Triatoma Proctacta* or American 'kissing bug'. Its bites are painless but can cause generalised itching, swelling, digestive symptoms and breathing problems.

Latex

Latex is the common name for the whitish, milky fluid that is produced by many plants, but it is the latex from the rubber tree *hevea braziliensis* that can cause anaphylaxis. Rubber trees are cultivated all over the world, but mainly in Malaysia. The latex is produced by making a diagonal cut in the bark of the tree and inserting a cup in which the fluid collects. After a few days the cup is emptied and moved to another cut in the bark.

Latex from the rubber tree is used in thousands of products. The one which is most likely to cause problems for people with anaphylaxis is rubber gloves. In anaphylaxis, the allergies associated with latex gloves are caused by natural impurities in the latex. These are called *extractable proteins*. These proteins are present in all natural latex products, but the amount of protein depends on how thoroughly the products have been washed during manufacture.

Latex allergies may begin locally but can, and do, lead to systemic anaphylaxis. If you have been sensitised to latex protein you are likely to react to any latex product and you are unlikely to grow out of it.

MANDY'S STORY

Mandy is allergic to latex, but it has taken her a very long time to realise this. There is atopy in her family: her uncle died of an asthma attack; her husband has mild psoriasis; and her daughter has asthma and eczema. Mandy suffers from asthma, eczema and hayfever.

She thinks her anaphylaxis began in 1990, on the day after the birth of her son. Mandy had a blood transfusion, and as she was given the fourth unit of blood she began to feel strange. Her body was itching and irritable, her tongue was swollen and tingly, and she had an asthma

---

attack. Mandy was given no explanation for this reaction.

As her son grew and Mandy entered the world of children's parties, she began to react to balloons and bouncy castles, but still she did not make the connection between the substance and her reactions. Finally in 1994 Mandy had an attack during a dental inspection: her face swelled up, her eyes misted over and she was wheezing badly.

Because of her eczema Mandy was already attending a dermatology clinic. When she told the nurse about these reactions, she was given a pair of latex-free gloves to take with her to the dentist. This she did, and the next check-up was uncomplicated.

However Mandy had still not realised the seriousness of her problem. In 1995 she reached into a children's 'party bag'. Unaware of its contents, she brushed a balloon within, and then rubbed her eye. Her face swelled, her eye closed, she was wheezing and shaking. Her husband telephoned the doctor who recommended taking ventolin and piriton. This made her sleep for a few hours, but when she awoke she found that her other eye was swelling and closing up. The doctor saw her, diagnosed an anaphylactic reaction, and prescribed adrenaline, which Mandy now carries everywhere with her in the form of an Epipen.

Mandy was tested and was found to be highly allergic to latex. She is also allergic to penicillin and eggs.

Avoiding contact with latex in everyday life can be surprisingly difficult. A hairbrush with a rubber handle, elastic in underwear, rubber-soled shoes – all these can provoke an immediate allergic reaction. Mandy also suspects that particles from rubber tyres which hang in the atmosphere in warm weather conditions set off her itching and wheezing. She cannot wear rubber gloves, and because she washes her hands frequently, they are always dry and sore.

But her attitude towards anaphylaxis is positive and optimistic. 'I have good and bad days,' she says. 'No one could understand this condition unless they had it. It's up to me to educate my friends and family, and to control my environment. Both my children understand how serious it is, and know what to do in an emergency. I have even persuaded the local ambulance men to flag my latex allergy on the paramedic computer – this means that, if I was in *any* emergency situation, the paramedics would know not to use latex gloves.

Rubber gloves are one of the most common causes of latex-induced anaphylaxis, but there are numerous other everyday items that contain latex. As Mandy observed, latex is not only all around us, it can even be in the air. Everyone encounters latex: babies suck on latex teats; it is in our clothing; in the mats in our cars; in erasers, balloons and elastic bands. Ironically enough, the increased use of condoms, to protect us from the threat of HIV infection, means that many more people are at risk of latex-induced anaphylaxis.

LATEX ALLERGIES IN HEALTHCARE WORKERS

Latex is used in numerous healthcare products, such as adhesive tape, elasticated bandages, enema tubing, mattresses, protective sheets, stomach tubes, urinary catheters, wound drains and, most frequently, gloves. Various reports have shown that 17 per cent of a sample of hospital employees regularly wear latex gloves, as do 38 per cent of dentists and up to 50 per cent of surgical and theatre staff.

The problems of healthcare workers becoming sensitised to latex have multiplied since the mid-1980s. This has happened because, since the worldwide spread of HIV and hepatitis, there has been a huge increase in the wearing of latex gloves. Before that, few healthcare workers – apart from those in the operating theatre – wore gloves.

The increased demand for gloves has led to an explosion in the number of gloves being manufactured. In 1987 there were 25 latex glove manufacturers in Malaysia; by 1990 there were over 400. Due to fierce competition between manufacturers, there have been attempts to cut costs, particularly by reducing the washing process.

In Britain, the National Health Service is supplied with 200 million pairs of gloves each year; 2.4 billion gloves are used annually in Europe, and 8.5 billion in the USA.

Latex also poses a threat to patients who are sensitised to it. The risks range from being examined by a dentist wearing latex gloves to undergoing surgery in which latex products are used.

ALLERGIC REACTIONS TO 'GLOVE POWDER'

It is often thought that the cornstarch powder used to make latex gloves easier to put on is an allergen, but this is not quite true. In fact there are two problems associated with glove powder. The first is that it can be a skin irritant, and thus make existing skin conditions worse. Secondly, allergens from the latex can stick to the powder and become airborne. This powder is then easily inhaled and can trigger an allergic reaction in anyone who has an atopic tendency.

LATEX AND FRUIT

When a substance causes an inflammatory reaction in our bodies, it is because it has been recognised, mistakenly, as a hostile factor. It is the *shape* of the proteins in the substance which set off the inflammatory response. Some of the proteins in latex have the same shape as some entirely different proteins that are present in certain fruits, including avocados, bananas, kiwi fruit, tomatoes, mangoes and chestnuts. Therefore a person whose anaphylaxis is triggered by latex may well have the same reaction to any of these fruits.

Other Causes

DRUGS

The drug which most commonly causes anaphylaxis is the antibiotic *penicillin*, particularly if it has been injected, rather than taken as tablets or medicine. However, anaphylaxis caused by penicillin is quite rare. If your doctor is about to prescribe penicillin he will usually ask if you are allergic to it. Many people have a reaction to this drug – for example they may feel nauseous or may even vomit. Simply reacting to a drug is *not* the same as having an anaphylactic reaction, although the effects of the reaction may appear similar to the early stages of anaphylaxis.

It is possible, though rare, to have an anaphylactic reaction to almost any drug. If you know that you are highly allergic to a particular drug, including those used in anaesthesia, you should ensure that anyone treating or prescribing for you also knows this.

EXERCISE

Physical exercise is a known cause of anaphylaxis. Some people are baffled by this because they are able to exercise quite safely most of the time. It may be the addition of some other factor, such as a particular food or even stress, which causes anaphylaxis when combined with exercise.

STRESS

As explained in Chapter 7, the effects of stress on our bodies are widespread and sometimes difficult to explain. Stress can bring about anaphylaxis, particularly if it is in combination with another known cause.

Idiopathic Anaphylaxis

This is the term used for anaphylaxis that does not seem to have any cause at all. Some people have been known to go into total anaphylactic shock, and no satisfactory explanation can be found for the attack. In many ways, idiopathy is the most frightening form of anaphylaxis. We will be looking at the implications of fear of anaphylaxis in Chapter 7.

To sum up, the causes of anaphylaxis are found in everyday factors that most of us encounter. These range from wasp stings to peanuts, from latex to stress, to nothing at all. Anaphylaxis can also be caused by very rare factors that only affect one or two individuals. For this reason, someone can be having an anaphylactic attack, but no one around them identifies it as such because there is no apparent cause. Nevertheless, if you know or are told that the person may have allergies, or if you see any of the known features of an anaphylactic attack, treat for anaphylaxis as quickly as you can (as described in Chapter 5). The message is: **if in doubt, treat**.

4

HOW TO RECOGNISE
ANAPHYLAXIS

It is vital to recognise an anaphylactic attack as early as possible in order to start life-saving emergency treatment. This may be difficult. The early features can be quite subtle and difficult to recognise. Or features may be very severe and could be mistaken for other medical emergencies. It will help if you are familiar with both the early features of anaphylaxis, and the features of a full-blown anaphylactic attack.

Early Features of Anaphylaxis

The early features of anaphylaxis can affect any part of your body. They may include:

* A tingling or burning sensation in your tongue and lips.
* Some difficulty in breathing due to tightness in your throat, larynx or chest.
* Small blisters appearing on your skin. You may also start itching all over, or become flushed.
* Sneezing, nose running, and your eyes becoming watery and itchy.
* Nausea and vomiting may develop.

30

- Feelings of foreboding and anxiety.

The early features of an anaphylactic attack vary. Some people experience most of these features. Other people may only experience one or two of them. If you are allergic to food, the most likely early features will be a tingling or burning sensation in your tongue or lips. If you are allergic to latex, the area of skin that is in contact with the latex is the first part that is likely to become red and blistered.

Features of Full-Blown Anaphylaxis

The early features of anaphylaxis do not always result in a full-blown anaphylactic attack, but they have the potential to do so. If a full-blown anaphylactic reaction develops, some of the early features of an anaphylactic reaction become more pronounced. These may include:

- Bloating of the tongue or lips; your tongue may become so swollen that it is too big for your mouth and sticks out.
- An increasing number of large red, raised weals begin to appear all over your body.
- Sensations of doom and fear. It is the effects of anaphylaxis on your airways and circulatory system which is particularly dangerous and people often have an innate sense of the danger that they face as a full-blown anaphylactic attack develops.
- The lining of the airways becomes increasingly swollen, thus narrowing the space through which oxygen can pass through to your blood. When the lining of the upper airways, the larynx and trachea, becomes swollen, there is a harsh rasping sound when you breathe in. This sound is called *stridor*. When the lining of the lower airways, the bronchi and bronchioles, becomes swollen, a sound like a feeble bagpipe can be heard when you breathe out. This is called a *wheeze*.

- In your circulatory system your blood vessels widen and become increasingly leaky. The volume of blood in your arteries, veins and heart is reduced, with the result that your pulse sounds fast but faint. This reduced blood supply leads to feeling faint, unconsciousness, and ultimately to shock and death.

Recognition of the features of full-blown anaphylaxis can make the difference between life and death.

DAVID'S STORY

In Chapter 3 we recounted the tragic death of Sarah, who died from anaphylaxis caused by eating crushed peanuts. Here Sarah's father, David, tells of the circumstances surrounding her death:

'The day Sarah died, she had been shopping alone for her mum's birthday present. She arrived home happily and began to wrap up the present in her bedroom. A few minutes later, she called out that she didn't feel well: she was wheezing and said her mouth felt funny. As her breathing became more and more difficult, my wife, Sarah's stepmother, decided to phone the doctor. Sarah had suffered asthma attacks for years, usually when a cold went to her chest, but she said this was strange, this was different. The doctor said take no chances, bring her in, but it was all too late. Sarah collapsed and died within minutes. I got the call at work.

'The irony was not lost. I'd worried for years about Sarah cycling on the main roads, her asthma, staying out late with her friends, drugs, drink, and all the usual things. How could I have foreseen that I would finally lose her to something as ludicrous as a small quantity of crushed peanut?

'But in the days following her death, the cause was a mystery. The paramedic on the scene said asthma, the hospital doctors agreed, but my wife challenged the diagnosis. She was there, she knew a simple asthma attack, she had suffered them herself for years. Finding out the truth became an obsession, because by not knowing we stood no chance of coming to terms with Sarah's death.'

David went on to discover that Sarah had unwittingly eaten crushed peanuts which were sprinkled on a piece of lemon meringue pie, and the cause of her death was later established as anaphylactic shock.

In the wake of his daughter's death David founded the Anaphylaxis Campaign, 'fighting for those with potentially fatal food allergies'. The Campaign now has over 4,000 members, acts as a highly effective lobby and has been instrumental in raising public awareness of anaphylaxis. The improvement in the ingredient information given on food packaging is just one of the successes attributable to the Anaphylaxis Campaign.

The Progress of Anaphylaxis

The initial features may precede a severe anaphylactic attack by only a minute or two, with almost no warning. However it may take up to an hour for a severe attack to develop.

Anaphylaxis may not progress beyond the early features. However, it is crucially important to recognise that a mild reaction has occurred, as re-exposure to the allergen which caused the reaction may cause a full-blown anaphylactic attack next time.

Here, you are in a position to take control and make a judgment. If you or someone close to you has an *atopic tendency* (suffers from asthma, eczema or hayfever or has these conditions in the family) and has experienced a mild reaction to a known cause of anaphylaxis, action must be taken.

ALISON'S STORY

Glynis ate a handful of salted nuts at the beginning of her pregnancy. She breast-fed baby Alison for nine months, occasionally eating a few peanuts. Alison suffered from dry skin, cradle-cap and then eczema, fairly badly. Glynis was encouraged to keep breast-feeding, as it might help to combat Alison's eczema. Along with countless other mothers, she treated her sore nipples with a breast cream which is now known to contain peanut oil. Arachis oil (peanut oil) and coconut oil were also contained in the skin creams prescribed for the baby. At the age of nine months Alison's eczema was so bad that she was admitted to hospital, and during this time she was weaned on to the bottle.

At the age of three Alison was given her first peanut, and suffered her first anaphylactic shock. She is now a normal, healthy nineteen-year-old who lives life to the full, and always carries piriton and adrenaline.

No-one knows exactly how and when Alison became sensitised to peanuts. Hindsight is a wonderful thing, but in the late 1970s there was very little awareness of the dangers of peanuts, even among healthcare professionals.

Other Conditions that Can Be Confused with Early Anaphylaxis

The early features of anaphylaxis are similar to those caused by a number of other conditions:

* Lip tingling can be caused by hyperventilation, which often accompanies panic attacks.

- Weals on the skin can be caused by contact with many noxious substances such as bleach.
- Sneezing and itching of the eyes may be caused by hayfever.
- Nausea and vomiting accompany a wide range of conditions, including food poisoning and pregnancy.

Other Conditions that Can Be Confused with Full-Blown Anaphylaxis

Even a full-blown anaphylactic attack can be mistaken for other medical conditions, particularly asthma and heart attacks.

BREATHING PROBLEMS AND ANAPHYLAXIS

Asthma and anaphylaxis can easily be confused. In an asthma attack, the lining of the lower airways swells up, causing the sufferer to wheeze as he breathes out. As the lining of the airways becomes more swollen, and breathing more laboured, a feature called recession develops. This is the in-drawing of flesh between the ribs and above the breastbone. When the asthmatic struggles to suck air into his lungs, recession becomes more marked.

Because anaphylaxis also involves swelling of the lining of the lower airways, a full-blown attack can appear almost identical to an acute asthma attack. In fact, it is thought that up to 15 per cent of all sudden deaths attributed to asthma are in fact caused by anaphylaxis.

In children particularly, inhalation of a foreign body, such as a bead, causes stridor and sometimes wheezing. This can appear very similar to an anaphylactic reaction.

HEART ATTACKS AND ANAPHYLAXIS

Usually, heart attacks are heralded by severe chest pain. However, they can sometimes occur with very little warning pain. When the person also goes into shock very suddenly, this kind of heart attack can easily be confused with an anaphylactic reaction. In addition, both heart attacks and anaphylactic reactions can be accompanied by stomach pain. This is another potential area of confusion.

Anaphylaxis can be one of the easiest or the most difficult conditions to accurately identify. **The key is to have good knowledge and awareness of the symptoms of anaphylaxis, and to be particularly aware of those people who are likely to suffer an anaphylactic attack.**
Anaphylaxis can be recognised from some or all of the following features:

- tingling or burning of the tongue and lips;
- tightness in the throat and larynx;
- blisters, redness and rashes on the skin;
- itching;
- sneezing and watery eyes;
- nausea and vomiting;
- feelings of anxiety and fear;
- swelling or bloating of the tongue or lips;
- breathing difficulties and wheezing;
- a rapid but faint pulse;
- fainting and unconsciousness.

They can vary in intensity, but any of these features should be taken seriously. If you suspect that a person is having an anaphylactic reaction, and adrenaline is available, inject him or her with adrenaline immediately (see Chapter 5) and seek medical help.

5

How to Treat an Anaphylactic Attack

As we have already seen, the main danger with anaphylaxis is that the inflammatory reaction can cause serious circulatory or breathing problems. This means that, within minutes, the person can go into shock or stop breathing. It is therefore crucial to stop, and then reverse, the effects of inflammation as quickly as possible. The main treatment for an anaphylactic attack is to inject adrenaline.

What is Adrenaline?

Adrenaline is a hormone that your body produces naturally from your adrenal glands, which are situated just above your kidneys. In fact we are all very familiar with the effects of adrenaline. If you have a fright, you become very pale or 'as white as a sheet'; your heart beats quickly; and you will often feel shaky. All these effects are caused by adrenaline. It is pumped into your bloodstream by the adrenal glands in response to your fear. The reason that you become very pale is because adrenaline causes the blood vessels in your skin to constrict, thus preventing the blood from colouring your skin. The blood is redirected to your muscles so you can either fight or run away; and the increased heart rate ensures that your muscles are well supplied with blood.

During other stressful situations, such as a full-blown anaphylactic attack, your adrenal glands pump large amounts of adrenaline into your bloodstream. Here, a critical balance between life and death develops. Adrenaline counteracts the inflammatory response by constricting the blood vessels and preventing them from becoming leaky.

However, if the inflammatory effects of the anaphylactic attack overwhelm the counteracting effects of adrenaline, the blood vessels become increasingly wide and leaky, leading to circulatory collapse or respiratory arrest. To treat a full-blown anaphylactic attack successfully, you have to ensure that the effects of the adrenaline outweigh the effects of the anaphylaxis. You can do this by introducing more adrenaline into the bloodstream.

What's the Best Way of Taking Adrenaline?

Adrenaline can be given in two ways, by injection or by inhalation. It cannot be taken by mouth (in tablet or medicine form) because it is a protein, and will thus be broken down in the gut and become ineffective. **The best way of taking adrenaline is by injecting it**.

The adrenaline enters the bloodstream quickly and, as long as you have positioned the needle reasonably well, you will receive the full dose. Adrenaline also enters the bloodstream quickly by inhalation, but many people find inhalers difficult to use, and so they may only receive a fraction of the intended dose.

There are a number of different injection systems available. The most basic system (despite being rather crude and unsatisfactory) is to have separate syringes, needles and small bottles or *phials* of adrenaline. You put the needle and syringe together, open the phial of adrenaline, work out the correct dosage, draw up the adrenaline into the syringe and then inject yourself. With a standard needle it is difficult to judge the correct depth for the injection. Moreover, in the midst of a full-blown anaphylactic attack, it would be difficult to carry out this complicated procedure.

The best injection systems have adrenaline, at the correct dosage, in pre-loaded syringes with needles that are pre-adjusted to the correct length. This means that in an emergency situation adrenaline can be delivered quickly, accurately and in the correct dosage. There are four preparations available: Epipen, Anapen, Min-I-Jet and Ana-Guard.

EPIPEN

To use the Epipen, remove the cap and push it against your outer thigh (see p. 40). This releases a spring-activated needle that delivers the pre-loaded adrenaline to the correct depth. Hold the device for at least 10 seconds against your thigh after the needle has been activated, allowing the full dose of adrenaline to be injected. If necessary, this device can be used through clothing. Epipen is pre-loaded with either an adult dose or a child's dose. Your doctor will prescribe whichever is appropriate.

ANAPEN

To use the Anapen, remove the black needle cap and the black safety cap from the firing button. Push the Anapen against your outer thigh and press the red firing button. This activates the spring-loaded needle, delivering the pre-loaded adrenaline to the correct depth. Hold the device against your thigh for at least 10 seconds to ensure that the full dose of adrenaline is injected. If necessary, this device can be used through clothing. Anapen is pre-loaded with either an adult dose or a child's dose. Your doctor will prescribe whichever is appropriate.

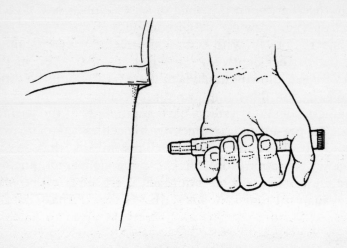

Injecting the Epipen into the outer thigh

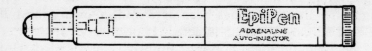

The Epipen

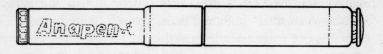

The Anapen

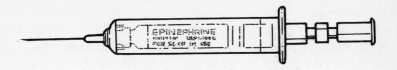

The Min-I-Jet

MIN-I-JET

To use the Min-I-Jet, first remove the protective caps from the injector and adrenaline phial. Now thread the phial into the injector for three-and-a-half turns, causing the needle to penetrate the stopper on the phial. Hold the device with the needle uppermost, and press the phial gently to remove any excess air. The Min-I-Jet is ready to use, and now you need to inject yourself in your outer thigh.

ANA-GUARD

To use the Ana-Guard, first remove the blue needle cover, hold the syringe upright and push the plunger to expel excess air and adrenaline. The plunger still stop automatically. Now rotate the rectangular plunger a quarter turn to the right, where it will align with a slot in the syringe. The Ana-Guard is ready to use, and now you need to inject yourself in your outer thigh. If necessary, the Ana-Guard can be used to give a second dose of adrenaline by turning the plunger a further quarter turn to the right. The dose that the Ana-Guard gives can be adjusted for children.

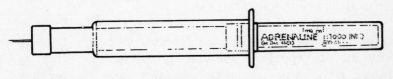

The Ana-Guard

With all of these devices, it is important that your doctor has shown you how to use them, and that you have been given the opportunity to practise with a dummy device. The Epipen and Anapen, with their spring-activated needles, are easier to use than the Min-I-Jet or Ana-Guard. The Epipen and Anapen do not require assembly and the person administering the medication does not need to be familiar with injection technique. These two factors could be crucial in an emergency situation. Also, Epipen and Anapen have longer shelf lives: two years as compared with six months for the other two devices.

ADRENALINE AND VERY YOUNG CHILDREN AND BABIES

The safe dose of adrenaline for babies and children under two is less than that contained in the junior pre-loaded syringe. Therefore you should not use one of these syringes for a child under two. However, anaphylactic reactions in children under two years old are extremely rare. If a child needs to have adrenaline available at this age, he or she would need to be under specialist care.

Inhaling Adrenaline

Inhaled adrenaline is given using a device called a metered dose inhaler (MDI). This is a sealed metal canister that sits inside a plastic holder. Adrenaline is mixed together with a propellant inside the metal canister.

As you press the metal canister down inside the plastic holder, the metering valve releases a precisely measured amount of propellant containing adrenaline. When you inhale at the same time as pressing the metal canister down, adrenaline is delivered onto the surface of the lungs where it is quickly absorbed into the bloodstream. Used correctly, adrenaline delivered by an MDI is an effective treatment for anaphylaxis, particularly for treating swelling in the airways.

To receive an adult dose of adrenaline, you need to take about 15 inhalations of adrenaline. For a child or baby, you will need to consult your doctor for the appropriate number of inhalations.

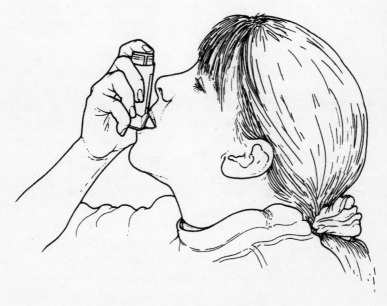

Using a metered dose inhaler (MDI)

However, most people, even when they are properly trained, do not use MDIs correctly. This means that we cannot be sure that all the adrenaline will reach the bloodstream. In a life-threatening situation, it is crucial that the adrenaline is reliably delivered. Even if a person can use an inhaler correctly, if they are very distressed, or even in a state of collapse, the MDI will be inadequate.

Side-Effects of Adrenaline

Adrenaline is a powerful drug and, even though it is surprisingly safe, it is not without its dangers. The most obvious side-effects are caused by the constriction of blood vessels, resulting in cold fingers, toes and a dry mouth. Adrenaline is also a stimulant, causing tremors and making the heart beat strongly and quickly. The danger is that it may over-stimulate your heart and actually stop it beating at all. People with heart problems are particularly vulnerable.

However, the danger from an anaphylactic attack is far greater than the danger from adrenaline. This means that if someone is having an anaphylactic attack, even if they have heart problems, the balance of risk is in favour of using adrenaline. If the person's heart should stop, then they will need to be revived using the resuscitation procedure described in detail on p. 51. If you have a heart problem or any other medical problems and need to carry adrenaline, discuss with your doctor any aspects of your situation that may need special consideration.

Corticosteroids

Your body naturally produces its own steroids called corticosteroids. Corticosteroids are produced, like adrenaline, by the adrenal glands. Corticosteroids are the body's natural anti-inflammatory agents. They prevent inflammation from developing in the first place, by inhibiting the effects of the white blood cells and by preventing the production of inflammatory mediators.

You can take corticosteroids in tablet form or by injection. The problem is that they take at least 24 hours to become effective. This is not very helpful for someone who is rapidly developing a full-blown anaphylactic reaction. However, corticosteroids may be used if you are admitted to hospital and it appears that your anaphylactic attack is going to take some time to subside.

SIDE-EFFECTS OF CORTICOSTEROIDS

Steroids have a bad image, and people are often concerned about the side-effects of using them. This is due to publicity about athletes abusing anabolic steroids. However, anabolic steroids are quite different from the corticosteroids which our bodies naturally produce. The long-term use of corticosteroids has many unpleasant side-effects, including skin thinning and weight gain. **Nevertheless, using corticosteroids appropriately for the short period needed to treat an anaphylactic attack is entirely safe.**

Antihistamines

Histamine is one of the inflammatory mediators released during an inflammatory reaction. Antihistamines inhibit the effects of histamine, helping to dampen down inflammation. Antihistamines in tablet form, such as triludan or piriton, are very effective in hayfever, but they are not effective in treating a full-blown anaphylactic attack.

However, antihistamines can help to lessen the severity of an anaphylactic attack. If, for example, you think you may have eaten a food that you are allergic to, taking an antihistamine tablet immediately may mean that you suffer a less serious anaphylactic reaction. It's therefore a good idea to carry a supply of antihistamine tablets, or antihistamine syrup for children, in case this situation occurs.

SIDE-EFFECTS OF ANTIHISTAMINES

Antihistamines are generally a very safe form of medication. Longer-established antihistamines may cause drowsiness, but with newer antihistamines, such as triludan, this is not usually a problem. As with any medication, there are one or two rare side-effects and a few drugs that should not be taken at the same time, so make sure you read the information supplied with the particular antihistamine that you intend to use.

Treating an Anaphylactic Attack

If you have previously experienced either the early features of anaphylaxis or a full-blown anaphylactic attack, and you suspect an anaphylactic reaction is developing, it is essential to act **immediately**. This means giving yourself an injection of adrenaline as soon as you experience any of the features of anaphylaxis. These could include lip tingling, tightness in the throat or even a sense of foreboding that an anaphylactic attack is about to occur. The sooner adrenaline is given, the easier it is to maintain a favourable balance between the life-threatening effects of the inflammation and the life-saving effects of adrenaline. **In order for you to be able to act promptly and be in control of an anaphylactic attack, it is essential to carry adrenaline on you at all times**.

After injecting adrenaline, you will usually experience considerable improvement in your condition within about 30 seconds. However, the effects of the adrenaline may wear off after 10–15 minutes. If this happens, and the symptoms of anaphylaxis reappear, you must then give yourself another injection of adrenaline. In fact, you may need a number of adrenaline injections, spaced apart by as little as 10 minutes. The only way you can be prepared for this is to **always carry at least two pre-loaded adrenaline injections**.

GETTING MEDICAL HELP

If a full-blown anaphylactic attack develops and you do need repeated injections of adrenaline, your supply can rapidly get used up. Even if you are only experiencing the early features of an anaphylactic attack, **you must seek professional medical help urgently**.

The best way of getting medical help will depend on where you live and the quality of the services available. If you live within 5–10 minutes of a hospital with a casualty department, someone should drive you there as soon as you have had your first dose of adrenaline.

If you live some distance from a casualty department, it may be best to phone for an ambulance and also to contact your doctor. Most ambulance crews carry adrenaline, and they have equipment to assist your breathing should this become necessary. Most doctors carry adrenaline, but often no more than one or two phials.

When telephoning for help, or when arriving at the casualty department, it is very important to impress upon the medical staff the urgency of the situation. You need to convey the message: '**This person is having a life-threatening anaphylactic attack.**'

If the anaphylactic attack is happening when you arrive in hospital you will almost certainly be given a 'drip'. This involves inserting a hypodermic needle into a vein, usually in your arm. A bag containing the drugs you need is attached to a tube, which leads into the other end of the hypodermic needle. In this way you can receive the drugs *intravenously*, or directly into the vein. If you are having difficulty breathing you will be given oxygen via a face mask. If you do not respond well to this treatment you may be taken to the intensive care unit which has the equipment needed to support your airways and circulatory system.

Once the anaphylactic attack has subsided, it is important that you are kept under observation in hospital for at least another four hours. This is because a second anaphylactic attack can occur shortly after the first one. A second attack is most likely to occur within four hours, although it can also occur after that time. The features of anaphylaxis have been known to last up to 20 days, so when you do return home you must have a supply of adrenaline with you, and preferably someone to watch over you for quite some time.

Questions Commonly Asked by People with Anaphylaxis

WHAT IF MY DOCTOR WILL NOT PRESCRIBE ADRENALINE FOR ME?

Unfortunately, some doctors are not as well informed about anaphylaxis as they should be. Your doctor may fail to meet your needs in a number of ways. Perhaps he will not prescribe the adrenaline in the delivery system you prefer (for example, the Anapen or the Epipen). Perhaps he will only prescribe one dose of adrenaline and none as a spare, or, if you are really unfortunate, he may not be willing to prescribe adrenaline at all.

If you experience any of these problems with your doctor, first try to explain the problem of anaphylaxis from your point of view. Maybe you could show your doctor this book! He may then be persuaded to reconsider your case.

If this approach does not work, your best option is to change doctors. If you ask around in your local community you will probably find other people with anaphylaxis – ask them who they think is the best doctor to see. Then all you have to do is to take your medical card to the new doctor's surgery and ask to be placed on his list. Your next step should be to make an appointment with him to ensure that he will offer the treatment you need.

WHAT IF I'M NOT SURE WHETHER AN ANAPHYLACTIC ATTACK IS OCCURRING?

Anaphylaxis can easily be confused with other conditions. In particular, anaphylaxis can be mistaken for hyperventilation, and a full-blown attack can seem like severe asthma or even a heart attack (see p. 35). It is therefore essential to have a good knowledge of anaphylaxis so that you can make an informed judgement. If someone appears to have anaphylaxis, and you know that they have had anaphylaxis before or you know that they have an atopic tendency, **you should assume that they are having an anaphylactic reaction**. In the heat of the moment, and if a person is in such a bad state that they cannot communicate, you may not be able to get confirmation from them. In such a situation, if you think someone is having an anaphylactic attack, you should treat that person for anaphylaxis. Or, to put it very simply, **if in doubt, treat**.

By taking such action, you may actually give someone adrenaline when they are not having an anaphylactic attack. Although using adrenaline carries some minimal risk, the risk is far higher if a person who is having an anaphylactic attack is left untreated.

WHAT IF I'M ASTHMATIC AND I'M BECOMING SHORT OF BREATH? SHOULD I USE MY RELIEVER INHALER?

If you are asthmatic and you are having an anaphylactic attack your chest may tighten just as it does when you have an asthma attack. If this happens, you can use your asthma reliever inhaler, for example ventolin, **in addition to** adrenaline. Your reliever inhaler is **not** a substitute for adrenaline.

WHAT IF I HAVE AN ANAPHYLACTIC REACTION AND I DON'T HAVE ANY ADRENALINE?

You must get adrenaline and professional medical help as quickly as possible. If you know that someone else carries adrenaline, borrow theirs. Call an ambulance or your doctor, or go straight to casualty – whichever option gives you the fastest access to adrenaline and professional medical help.

WHAT IF THE ADRENALINE I'M CARRYING IS OUT OF DATE?

If this is the only adrenaline you have and you are having an anaphylactic attack, then some adrenaline is better than none. However, if your adrenaline is more than about *three* months past its expiry date it is almost useless. In addition, check the colour of the adrenaline. It should be clear, like water. If it has a yellow or brown discolouration, or particles floating in it, it should not be used.

Questions Commonly Asked by Carers

AFTER I HAVE GIVEN ADRENALINE, AND I'M WAITING FOR HELP TO ARRIVE, WHAT SHOULD I DO?

Keep the person as calm and as comfortable as possible. If they are cold, put a light blanket around them. If they are thirsty, give them sips of water.

WHAT IF THE PERSON HAS ALREADY STOPPED BREATHING?

If the person is having an anaphylactic attack, is no longer breathing and is without a pulse, then you must resuscitate him (see below). You must also give adrenaline if it has not been given in the last 10 minutes.

Resuscitation

If a person has collapsed and appears not to be breathing, and also seems to be without a pulse, there are a number of steps you must follow:

HOW TO TREAT AN ANAPHYLACTIC ATTACK

1. Turn the person onto his back, ensuring he is on a firm survace.
2. Lift the chin forward with the index finger and middle finger of one hand, and press the forehead backwards with the heel of the other hand. This prevents the tongue from blocking the airway.
3. Check if the person is breathing by placing your ear above his nose or mouth and looking along the chest and abdomen. If he is breathing, you will feel his breath on your face and see his chest or abdomen moving.
4. If he is not breathing, turn his head to one side, and pass a finger around inside his mouth to make sure there are no obstructions such as vomit or false teeth. Remove any obvious obstructions. Do not push your fingers down his throat.
5. Re-check for breathing. If he is still not breathing, you must start mouth-to-mouth ventilation, inflating the collapsed person's lungs using your own breath. Keeping the forehead pressed back with one hand, use the thumb and forefinger of this hand to pinch the person's nose. With the other hand keep his chin lifted forwards. Take a breath in, then seal your lips around the collapsed person's lips and breathe out slowly. As you breathe into the person's mouth, you will see his chest rise. Remove your mouth, and the elastic recoil of his lungs will cause him to breathe out automatically. Inflate the person's lungs for a second time and re-check to see if he has started breathing.
6. Now check to see if the person has a pulse. To do this, feel for the *carotid* pulse with your fingertips by sliding your fingers sideways from the voice box (Adam's Apple) to the hollow between the voice box and adjacent muscle. Feeling for a pulse at the wrist is unreliable under these circumstances.
7. If there is no pulse you must start chest compressions. First, find the point where the bottom of the ribs meets the breast bone. Then place the heel of one hand two finger breadths above this point, and interlock your other

hand on top. With your weight directly above your hands, and your arms straight, press down vertically to move the breast bone 1½-2 inches (4–5cm). The movement should be smooth and firm, not jerky. When you release the pressure from the breast bone, without removing your hands, the chest wall will rise again.

8. If the person has a pulse but is not breathing, you need only perform mouth-to-mouth ventilation. If the person is without a pulse, you will always need to perform mouth-to-mouth ventilation and chest compressions together. If you are by yourself, proceed in a cycle of two mouth-to-mouth ventilations followed by 15 chest compressions. Ideally, two people will perform resuscitation together, one person being responsible for chest compressions, and the other for mouth-to-mouth ventilation. For every five chest compressions there should be one mouth-to-mouth ventilation, delivered just after the fifth compression as the chest is expanding. You will ideally achieve 80 chest compressions a minute.

If a person has had an anaphylactic attack it is unlikely that you will be able to restore his pulse and breathing. This is very much a holding operation until professional help arrives. If you do manage to restore the person's breathing, place the person on their side, rolled slightly forward with the position maintained by the person's bent top leg. The head should be tilted backwards to keep the airway open. This is called the recovery position. Observe carefully until help arrives.

RESUSCITATING INFANTS AND SMALL CHILDREN

For infants and small children, again ensure they are on a firm surface, pull the chin forward and check for breathing. If there is no breathing, gently clear the mouth of any obstruction using a finger. Be very careful not to touch the back of the throat of an infant or a child. Infections can cause swelling of the back of the throat which car be exacerbated if touched, causing complete blockage of the airway.

In an infant, place your mouth over his mouth and nose, and inflate the lungs sufficiently to cause the chest to rise. Allow the chest to fall, and repeat five times.

Now check for a pulse. In an infant the best pulse is the *brachial* pulse. This is found on the inside of the arm, midway between the shoulder and the elbow. Press gently against the bone using your index and middle fingers. If there is no pulse you will need to start chest compressions.

In an infant the correct place to press is the upper part of the breast bone. This is found by drawing an imaginary line between the nipples. Place the tips of two fingers just below the mid-point of this line. Press here to a depth of 2cm. Give five compressions for every ventilation, achieving 100 compressions and 20 ventilations a minute.

For a child below school-age, find the correct position to press on the chest as for an adult. Press with just one hand, moving the chest 3cm. As for an infant, give five compressions for every ventilation, achieving 100 compressions and 20 ventilations per minute. For a larger child, the technique is the same as for an adult.

Everyone would benefit from being taught to give artificial respiration in a First Aid class, rather than having to make their first attempt during a real-life emergency. In Britain the St John's Ambulance, St Andrew's Association and the British Red Cross all run First Aid courses. More information on how to contact them is in Useful Addresses.

6

LIVING WITH ANAPHYLAXIS

It is difficult to cope with knowing that you, or someone near you, may have an anaphylactic attack. By definition, anaphylaxis is frightening. The speed at which an attack can take hold is alarming, as are the physical changes which affect the person having the attack. Yet there are ways to cope with having the condition in your life.

There are very few of us whose health is perfect and whose bodies are in complete working order. Perhaps you are short-sighted, asthmatic, diabetic, suffer from hayfever, epilepsy or back pain. These are all conditions which people have to endure. They seldom go away **but they can be controlled**. The short-sighted person controls his condition by wearing glasses or contact lenses, the asthmatic uses inhalers, the diabetic takes insulin, and so on. We try not to let these conditions dominate our lives; we learn to live with them. Like these other conditions, anaphylaxis does not bother you all the time, but you need to be aware of it and take the necessary precautions.

In an ideal world the best way to deal with anaphylaxis would be always to avoid anything that triggers it. Unfortunately, in the real world, this is not always possible. The best option is to find ways of minimising the likelihood of an attack while living a normal life. And, in the words of novelist Susan Hill, who suffers from anaphylaxis, 'We are lucky. We know what is wrong with us, and we can carry our life-saving equipment around with us.'

One of the most effective ways of avoiding your trigger is to tell as many people as you can about your anaphylaxis, and about what causes it. If those around you are aware of your problem, they are likely to keep the triggers away from you. However they will not be infallible, so you still need to remain vigilant and in control of the situation.

In this chapter we look at how to identify and avoid the common triggers of anaphylaxis, and investigate ways of controlling the condition.

Identifying the Trigger

When someone has had an anaphylactic attack, they need to be sure what triggered the attack so they can try and avoid that trigger. In 1994 the British government's Chief Medical Officer (CMO) issued clear guidelines to doctors in a document called the CMO's Update. This document says that: 'All patients suspected to suffer from peanut allergy should be referred to a specialist clinic. Even if the diagnosis is in doubt, patients should on no account be advised to test their reaction by eating peanuts ...'

If your doctor is unable to find an allergy clinic, he can look one up in the handbook issued by the British Society for Allergy and Clinical Immunology. Entitled *National Health Service Allergy Clinics*, the handbook lists the addresses of the allergy clinics, their areas of expertise (for example, hayfever, allergic asthma, anaphylaxis, allergy to insect stings), and the names of the consultants or senior medical practitioners who run them. (See Useful Addresses, p. 97)

In Britain if you have a suspected severe food allergy and are referred to an allergist you will probably see her at your local hospital. First of all you will be asked about your medical history and that of members of your family. In particular the allergist will be looking for evidence of an atopic tendency. She will want to know what you think may have caused your problem, how much of the suspected allergen you consumed and how serious your reaction was.

You may be given a medical examination and then a skin test. This involves putting a few drops of a highly diluted solution of the allergen on the skin, and then scratching the skin's surface so that the weak substance leaks under the skin. After about 15 minutes the allergist will examine the testing area and see if there has been a reaction, and if so how severe it is. The stronger your skin's reaction, the more severe the allergy.

The allergist may also give you a blood test to see if you have antibodies to the substance in your blood. If these results suggest that you are likely to have an anaphylactic reaction to, say, peanuts, you will probably be prescribed one or two injections of adrenaline, and told to keep the pre-loaded syringes with you at all times. You may also be prescribed inhaled adrenaline and oral antihistamines.

Radio Allergo Sorbent Test (RAST)

This test is used to see if you have any antibodies against a specific allergen in your blood. A sample of the allergen is attached to a suitable surface such as a paper disc. A sample of your plasma (blood without red blood cells) is then passed over the paper disc. If you have any antibodies against the allergen, they will now attach to the allergen. The next stage is to pass a special radioactive label through the paper disk that will only attach to your antibodies. If you have antibodies to the allergen, the paper disc will now be radioactive, if you do not have antibodies to the allergen, the paper disc will not be radioactive.

The allergy nurse will show you how to use the injection, and explain when and how to take the rest of the prescribed medication.

Avoiding Trigger Foods

In Chapter 3, we stressed the importance of avoiding feeding your unborn child or young baby with known food allergens, such as peanuts. But what do you do if your baby is allergic to milk? There are some baby milks on the market which have been *hydrolysed*, or processed to reduce the size of the protein molecules which most often cause an allergic response. Hydrolysed milk has been around for over 50 years, and in Britain some of the most well-known baby milk companies produce it. Most high street pharmacists stock it, although it may not be on display. The milk, which is quite expensive, is available over the counter or on prescription.

In order to avoid eating certain foodstuffs ourselves, we need to know if they are in our food. With fresh, home-prepared food this is simple: you do not buy the offending food, you do not cook with it, and you do not eat it. With food that is pre-packaged or bought from a food outlet it is not so simple. Many of the problems arise because the food is labelled, or described, misleadingly.

FOOD LABELLING

By law the food that we buy in shops must display a list of ingredients. Assuming you know that your particular allergen may be listed under another name (for example, 'ground nuts' instead of peanuts), and assuming that you have read the labels diligently, you might think you are safe. Unfortunately, this is untrue. You may still be buying a life-threatening portion of the offending foodstuff, and yet have absolutely no idea. The reason for this is the 25 per cent rule.

THE 25 PER CENT RULE

In Britain, the current food labelling regulations say that any ingredient which makes up less than 25 per cent of the whole product does not have to be broken down into its constituent ingredients and have each of those ingredients listed. An example of this could be a slice of salami on a pizza. So small amounts of an allergen may be omitted from the ingredients list. However, many supermarkets and shops have undertaken to provide this information even though it is not legally required. The regulations are currently under review, and it may well be that soon even the merest trace of a known anaphylaxis trigger will have to be identified on the food label.

Many British shops and supermarkets are aware of the dangers associated with food allergies. Some produce leaflets listing those of their products which do not contain particular ingredients or combinations of particular ingredients; some keep a mailing list of people with food allergies so they can be informed about the content of new products. The power wielded by the big supermarkets can also be employed to persuade suppliers to remove certain ingredients from their products. Supermarkets with in-store bakeries are aware of the dangers of *cross-contamination*, and so they warn us, for example, that traces of nuts may inadvertently drift from the Danish pastries to the brown loaves.

It is largely due to pressure from people concerned about anaphylaxis that these steps have been taken. In order to continue raising awareness of anaphylaxis this pressure needs to be maintained. This could be done by writing to shops and asking which of their products contain, say, sesame seeds, or which non-dairy foods include added milk protein. You could request, for example, that an area of the in-store bakery be protected from the possibility of cross-contamination so that you, too, could enjoy freshly baked bread.

KOSHER FOOD LABELLING

Kosher food is prepared in accordance with Jewish dietary laws. In Britain, kosher certification is under the jurisdiction of the Kashrut Division of the London Beth Din (law court). Meat products comply with the general UK laws on food labelling, except that the product is additionally identified as kosher. The product will have been prepared under kosher rules from the abattoir right through to the finished consumer pack.

Non-meat products similarly comply with UK regulations, with special emphasis on the separation of dairy products and meat products. So food that is labelled as a dairy product will not contain any animal source ingredients whatsoever. This scrutiny will be far-reaching: for example, cooking oil which has previously been used for cooking meat products could not be used to cook kosher food. Phosphates, a food ingredient, can be from an animal or mineral source under UK regulations, but under kosher rules they can only be from minerals.

Eggs are considered 'neutral', neither dairy nor meat, and so are not restricted in kosher food, although pasteurised eggs tend to be used.

Peanuts are allowed under Jewish law, so traces of peanut are not especially mentioned on kosher labelling.

If you are allergic to animal products you would be extremely safe with kosher food. The checks and restrictions which are applied before kosher certification is granted are so tough that many products which are labelled as vegetarian – and therefore should not contain meat – could not be labelled as kosher.

Food Additives

This is another area of concern for people with food allergies. Food additives are deliberately added to food during processing. Their main purposes are to preserve it longer, stop bacteria and mould developing, and prevent the food from 'going off'. They can improve the taste, texture and colour of food, and even its nutritional value.

Nevertheless many people are sceptical about the benefits of food additives, including those additives which are approved for use by the European Union – those denoted by E-numbers. Many people, especially children, react strongly to various food additives, particularly E102 (tartrazine) and E210 (benzoic acid). It is possible to get a comprehensive list of food additives from the Ministry of Agriculture, Fisheries and Food (see Useful Addresses).

The Food Intolerance Databank

This databank holds detailed information about foods that are known to cause allergic reactions, and lists foods that are free from those ingredients. The databank is currently based on the following ingredients:

- **Milk and milk derivatives**
- **Egg and egg derivatives**
- **Wheat and wheat derivatives**
- **Soya and soya derivatives**
- **BHA and BHT** – These are antioxidants, which stop fatty foods from going rancid. BHA is listed on food labels as E320, and can be found in beef stock cubes and cheese spread. BHT is listed as E321, and can be found in chewing gum.
- **Sulphur dioxide** – This is a preservative, found in foods containing E221–E227 inclusive.

- **Benzoates** – These are preservatives, found in foods containing E210–E219 inclusive.
- **Azo colours** – This is a group of colours including E102 (tartrazine – found in soft drinks), E110 (sunset yellow – found in biscuits), E122, E123, E124, E128 (red – found in sausages), E151 (black), E154 (brown – found in kippers), E155 (chocolate brown) and E180.

Due to the current uncertainty about whether or not refined peanut oil contains peanut allergen, the data-bank does not issue 'peanut-free' or 'contains peanut' lists, although it hopes to produce such lists in the future. Also, some of the major supermarket chains do not supply the Databank with information about ingredients, but publish their own lists which are freely available to the public.

Access to information in the Databank is only via a registered dietician. If you feel you would benefit from having some of these lists, you should ask your doctor to refer you to a dietician, who can then request the lists for you (see Useful Addresses).

Most hospitals in Britain have a state-registered dietician on the staff. Dieticians can also be found within health centres or community hospitals, and some are in private practice. Until very recently, it was only possible to see a dietician if you were referred by a doctor or medical practitioner. Now, new guidelines issued for state-registered dieticians (of which there are over 4,000 in Britain) mean that members of the public can contact them direct. The dietician must get confirmation of the patient's condition from his or her doctor, and inform the doctor about the dietary changes which have been suggested.

VISITING A DIETICIAN

If you have had an anaphylactic reaction to food, it is likely that you will know what has caused it. For example, if your allergy is to milk, your dietician will advise you on how to avoid milk and milk products. She will give you lists of manufactured foods containing milk, and show you how milk may be described in different ways on food labels. Your dietician will tell you where to get recipes for milk-free cooking, and will probably suggest that you focus on home-cooked food using basic ingredients.

Having made the necessary changes to your daily diet, your dietician will want to ensure that you are getting getting adequate nutrition for your growth and well-being. You will be shown alternative sources of nutrition and may be advised to take vitamin or mineral supplements. It is important to establish a manageable and varied diet, particularly for children, so that they will be happy to stick to it. In the case of a child, he or she must be involved as early as possible, so as to be alert to the dangers, and to understand the importance of avoiding these foods. Always keep a close check on the eating habits of food-anaphylactic children.

You may be put in touch with a health visitor with a special interest in food allergies who will be able to offer support and encouragement. And you will probably be asked to return to the clinic in about two months' time, when your weight and growth may be checked to ensure that you are still getting sufficient nutrition.

EATING OUT

Restaurants, cafés, bars and diners are a few steps behind shops in responding to the needs of people with anaphylaxis. In Britain you are unlikely to be handed a leaflet itemising the ingredients of your gourmet meal, although in Canada certain restaurants choose to supply ingredient lists and have a member of staff available to answer questions about the content of each dish.

When eating out, the onus is very much on the person with anaphylaxis. Meekly explaining to a waiter that you are allergic to peanuts may not be adequate; the waiter could well be a temporary member of staff who does not know the procedure for checking the content of dishes, or he may be too busy (or too lazy) to check properly. You must impress upon the *person in charge* that if you eat even a trace of peanut you could die right there in the restaurant.

THE CATERING INDUSTRY

Nearly everyone who dies from food-induced anaphylaxis dies as a result of having eaten something away from home. This, coupled with the fact that the number of people with severe food allergies is rising with each generation, should be enough to worry the catering industry into tightening up on procedures. Or, as one lady, who has had severe anaphylactic attacks as a result of unknowingly eating nuts, put it: 'We have to treat nuts in kitchens almost as a poison.'

So far, the catering industry has not been as quick as the food retailing industry to understand and respond to the needs of people with anaphylaxis.

In Britain an initiative undertaken by the Anaphylaxis Campaign has led to the rewriting of standards for the National Vocational Qualifications (NVQs). Similar action has been taken with the Scottish Vocational Qualifications (SVQs). These are nationally recognised qualifications.

The revised standard, which will be part of the NVQ and SVQ catering training from January 1997, covers adoption and implementation of a code of practice for avoiding and dealing with anaphylaxis; understanding the dangers of consuming food containing potent allergens; and understanding the necessity for rigorous preparation and serving procedures, and the need to provide accurate information about ingredients.

Of course, not everyone in the catering industry will have these qualifications. There are, however, a few obvious precautions which could be taken, and which could become the basis of a company anaphylaxis protocol:

- Staff must be taught about anaphylaxis – how it happens, what causes it and how serious it can be. The Anaphylaxis Campaign (see Useful Addresses) can provide an information sheet.
- If nuts or other common triggers of anaphylaxis are used in a recipe, this information must be passed all the way down the line to the serving staff.
- If possible, replace known triggers of anaphylaxis with other ingredients.
- If non-nut oil has previously been used to cook nut products it must now be viewed as a trigger.
- Ensure that chefs, cooks and food-handlers read the ingredients lists on foods that are bought in from suppliers.
- If using known triggers in food preparation, take stringent steps to avoid cross-contamination during preparation and service.

TAKING THE FIRST STEPS

Hilton National has 25 hotels across Great Britain. Following a food and beverage review, ingredients of all dishes offered in every restaurant have been collated and listed. Every kitchen works from an 'ingredients bible', and the chefs do not deviate from the agreed ingredients for each dish. Every menu is printed with the following: *For allergy sufferers, we will be more than happy to provide you with details of the ingredients for each dish. Please ask your waiter.*

In the county of Hereford and Worcester, the Trading Standards Service set out to find which of the restaurants, cafés and take-aways in the region were anaphylaxis-aware. Of the 53 premises checked, only 36 per cent told customer about the presence of nuts or nut products in the foods available. The service, which now issues information about anaphylaxis to local businesses, also wants legislation to make declaration of nuts and nut products in food compulsory.

EATING ON JOURNEYS

With a little preparation and forward planning, it is possible to avoid certain foods during journeys. The simplest solution is to take your own food with you. If you are intending to eat on an aircraft, ferry or train, it is advisable to let them know of your anaphylaxis beforehand so that they can provide suitable meals.

British Airways, for example, encourages passengers to inform them of food allergies in advance. This is particularly important with children, for if the child is travelling alone, or if the parent is elsewhere in the aircraft when the cabin staff come by, he or she might be offered some peanuts or other food likely to cause an attack.

When you reach your destination, remember that the well-known item of food which you can happily eat at home because you know it does not contain your allergen, may be produced overseas using different methods and could therefore be less safe to eat. This is particularly true of some well-known chocolate bars, which are manufactured under licence overseas and may not adhere to such strict production controls.

TRANSLATIONS

The Anaphylaxis Campaign and the British Allergy Foundation (see Useful Addresses) have produced two sets of translations, in many languages. One set explains that you have severe food allergies, and that you will become ill if you eat certain foods. The other set contains information about what you need other people to do should an anaphylactic attack occur. These translations are available free to members.

Avoiding Latex

Avoiding latex in everyday life is probably harder than avoiding peanuts or any of the other offending foods. Latex is everywhere, and its presence does not have to be announced on a label. Since it is used in over 40,000 different products, latex is obviously not going to go away; we need it too much.

LATEX-FREE CONDOMS

At present, condoms are manufactured from latex. Some types of condoms may have a reference to *allergy* in their name, but this is to do with whether or not they incorporate spermicidal lubricant, to which some people are allergic. The LIG Group has developed a polyurethane condom which is being tested in the USA and will be available in the future.

However, there are a few simple precautions you *can* take, such as not wearing rubber gloves for washing up, or carrying a pair of non-latex gloves with you when you go for a dental or medical examination. In Britain, Boots, the high street chemist, sells 'allergenic' gloves which are made from PVC (polyvinyl chloride, a synthetic material), and some of the big supermarket chains sell disposable vinyl household gloves. It is also possible to buy latex-free industrial-strength gloves. See the Useful Address section for more information on where to obtain latex-free gloves.

Perhaps you could follow Mandy's example (p. 24), and ask your local ambulance service to register details of your latex allergy on their computer, so that if you ever received emergency medical treatment the paramedics would avoid bringing you into contact with latex. Further reassurance for anyone with anaphylaxis could come from wearing the MedicAlert emblem.

MEDICALERT

MedicAlert is for people with medical conditions that are not necessarily apparent but which may well be life-threatening – these would include asthma, heart conditions and anaphylaxis. It is an international charity which provides personal medical information to medical staff in order to save lives.

Each member wears the MedicAlert emblem, either as a bracelet or a necklace. On the back of the emblem is a short description of their condition, guidance on treatment, a membership number and a 24-hour emergency telephone number. On telephoning this number and quoting the patient's identification number, the doctor or nurse is given additional medical information, the name of the patient's doctor and contact numbers for family members. This information has been supplied to MedicAlert by the patient and verified by his doctor.

MedicAlert operates in 43 countries and has four million members worldwide. Currently, in Britain, it costs £30 to join MedicAlert plus an annual fee of £8. (For details see Useful Addresses.)

LATEX AVOIDANCE FOR HEALTHCARE WORKERS

In the USA much has been done to protect both patients and healthcare workers from the problems associated with latex allergies. Workers can be screened for possible latex allergies, there are 'latex-free' areas, and many hospitals have their own latex protocols. In 1993 the American Food and Drug Administration announced that all medical devices containing latex had to carry a warning on the packet – 'this product contains natural rubber latex'. In Canada the medical authorities are considering labelling latex products, and are researching latex sensitivity in a large sample of healthcare workers.

In Britain the Department of Health set up a working group to examine the problem of latex sensitivity, and subsequently issued a bulletin entitled *Latex Sensitivity in the Health Care Setting*. Among the bulletin's conclusions are the need for more awareness about latex sensitisation among regulators, manufacturers, suppliers, purchasers, users of latex gloves and healthcare managers. There are no figures available on how many British healthcare workers are affected by latex sensitivity. See Useful Addresses for information on how to obtain this bulletin.

There are some measures which could be taken to lessen the likelihood of healthcare workers having anaphylactic reactions to latex. These include:

• Buying synthetic sterile surgical gloves which do not contain latex. (However some healthcare workers find that these are too restrictive for the precise finger movements they need to make in the course of their work.)

- Persuading manufacturers to publish the quantity of extractable latex proteins used in their products, and circulating these details to buyers of hospital supplies.
- Setting a maximum acceptable level of extractable proteins, and only buying gloves which are below that level.
- Health authorities committing to providing low-allergen or latex-free products.
- Healthcare workers being discouraged from wearing latex gloves unless it is really necessary. (This would be difficult in Britain because, at present, there are no published guidelines available as to which gloves should be worn in which situation.)

From a financial point of view it would be difficult at present to justify implementing these measures. Certainly more research is needed into the extent of the problem amongst healthcare workers, particularly those in Britain.

WHAT DOES 'HYPOALLERGENIC' MEAN?

Products marketed as being 'good for' people with allergies are sometimes labelled 'hypoallergenic'. This word simply means 'less allergenic', and is therefore fairly meaningless unless it goes on to explain exactly how much of the allergen the product contains. The American Food and Drug Administration has banned the use of the word 'hypoallergenic' on all medical devices containing latex, and has instead insisted on a prominent latex warning on the package.

Avoiding Insect Stings

Try avoiding wasps on a sunny afternoon when you are having lunch in the garden, or on the beach when you go to put a pile of sticky ice-cream wrappers in the litter bin – you cannot. Try avoiding bees if you are a bee keeper – you cannot. Avoiding being stung sometimes seems an impossible task, especially as many of us who have been stung did not even see the wasp until we felt the pain of the sting. Yet if you live completely at the mercy of wasps you have relinquished control of your life, and the wasp, or your fear of it, has won.

There are some simple steps you can take to lessen the likelihood of being stung. The following check list has been drawn up by people who are sensitised to wasp venom, and who know how dangerous their next sting could be:

- Never go barefoot anywhere, not even indoors.
- Never put on shoes or slippers without shaking them out first.
- If you find a wasps' nest near your home, have it removed or treated immediately. (In Britain, some councils' pest control departments will give priority to people with anaphylaxis, so it is worth mentioning this when you ring them.)
- Do not wear brightly coloured or patterned clothes outdoors.
- Do not wear perfume.
- If a wasp starts buzzing around you, do not start flapping your arms.
- Wear a hat and cover your arms and legs when you are in the garden.
- Keep doors and windows closed during the summer months. In America it is possible to buy custom-made frames covered with insect-proof mesh, which slot inside your window frames and enable you to leave the windows open without fear of insects flying in. When the wasp

season is over they are either removed from the windows and stored until next year, or they can be fitted permanently. These frames do not appear to be commercially available in Britain, but could be purpose-built by a joiner.

- Do not go fruit picking in the autumn – the ripe apple orchard really is no place for someone with anaphylaxis.
- Keep plenty of anti-wasp aerosol sprays around the house.

WHAT IF YOU DO GET STUNG?

If you are stung by a bee, remove the sting quickly. The advice on removing bee stings has been revised recently, following a new American study. We used to be told to pinch the sting out, preferably with tweezers, so as to prevent more venom pulsing out. The new advice is to quickly scrape the sting out with whatever is immediately available – perhaps a knife or a credit card. It is the *speed* of removal of the sting rather than the method that is critical. (This method only applies to bees, wasps do not leave their sting.)

Always carry your adrenaline with you and keep it by your bedside at night.

Desensitisation Treatment for Insect Sting Anaphylaxis

For some people, it's simply too difficult to live with the risk of having an anaphylactic reaction to a sting. For these people, it may well be worth investigating the possibility of being immunised against wasp or bee venom. There are a few venom immunotherapy clinics in Britain, and the treatment they offer is called *desensitisation* (making the patient less sensitive to the cause of their allergic reaction).

Professor David Warrell is Professor of Tropical Medicine

and Infectious Diseases at the University of Oxford and Consultant-in-Charge of the venom clinic at the Churchill Hospital in Oxford. His particular area of interest is the direct effects of animal venom: snake bites, spider bites, jellyfish stings, and scorpion, wasp and bee stings. While working with snake bite victims in the Tropics he witnessed several hundred anaphylactic attacks; this is because the only effective treatment for snake bites is to inject a potent anti-venom which has the side-effect of triggering anaphylaxis in up to 80 per cent of patients. His interest in venom and his experience in treating anaphylaxis led to him taking on the venom clinic in 1986.

In Britain there are only a handful of clinics offering desensitisation for patients with acute allergies. In order to receive the treatment, patients need a referral from their doctor. Professor Warrell also sees patients who have been brought into the casualty department. There are several hundred patients currently registered with the venom clinic, and he expects to see three or four new cases each week.

WHO CAN BE TREATED?

Not every patient who has severe sensitisation to bee or wasp stings will be suitable for the desensitising programme. Children are rarely treated, because it is likely that they will grow out of their sensitivity. Neither are pregnant women, because the treatment could provoke painful contractions of the uterus, one of the early features of anaphylaxis. And this could carry a slight risk of causing a miscarriage.

Then there are some people who cannot cope with the idea of the treatment: perhaps they cannot undertake the commitment to travel and attend the clinic; they may be frightened of injections; or they may be frightened of what they are being injected with.

Those who seem suitable for treatment are then tested for sensitivity to wasp or bee venom, using either the RAST test or skin prick testing as described on p. 56.

Desensitisation involves injecting the patient with a weak extract of venom. The strength of the injection is increased over a period of time, so that the patient can gradually build up tolerance to the venom. Treatment is usually continued for at least three years. A standard course of injections involves eight consecutive weekly injections, followed by a maintenance injection initially at four-weekly intervals. If that is tolerated well, the gap between the maintenance injections would be extended to five weeks, then six weeks, and so on, up to a three-month gap. Levels of antibodies against the allergen usually fall during the period of desensitisation. Most patients reach a point of being able to tolerate the equivalent of two wasp stings without reacting either locally or systemically by the end of the first eight weeks of desensitisation.

Using these modern venom preparations, patients who have been desensitised for three years have a more than a 90 per cent chance of being cured of their sensitivity.

Professor Warrell concedes that the experts do not really know how desensitisation works. 'The venom clinic is a marvellous exercise in preventive medicine, and there is overwhelming evidence that it *does* work,' he says. 'But I would like to be able to measure something related to the process of desensitisation.'

Even when patients have been desensitised, Professor Warrell still advises them to carry adrenaline. This is because in some people the effectiveness of the desensitising treatment can wear off over a number of months or years. In Professor Warrell's vast experience of anaphylaxis, adrenaline is '*the* life-saving drug'. He stresses the importance of the patient understanding when, and how, to use the adrenaline injection. 'A patient who is having an anaphylactic attack can lose consciousness within 30 seconds, so they must have their adrenaline immediately,' he insists.

Professor Warrell has seen many anaphylactic attacks and yet he does not want to frighten people unnecessarily. He remains impressed by the body's own ability to cope with this type of emergency. 'Considering the severity and speed of an anaphylactic reaction,' he says, 'it's amazing how few people die ...'

As we have seen, by following common sense trigger avoidance measures, and always carrying adrenaline with you, the risks of having an anaphylactic attack can be reduced to a fairly manageable level. Even so, anaphylaxis remains a worrying condition and the psychological effects on sufferers and their families should not be under-estimated. The next chapter looks at these effects more closely and suggests ways in which they can be alleviated.

7

THE PSYCHOLOGICAL
EFFECTS OF
ANAPHYLAXIS

As we have seen, there is much that can be done to limit exposure to the causes of anaphylaxis, and there is effective medication to treat the physical symptoms. But what about the psychological and emotional impact of the condition? It is very important to understand the impact anaphylaxis can have, and how seriously it can affect a person's life as well as that of his or her family.

We need to consider the emotional and physical symptoms experienced following an anaphylactic attack and, if the person who has experienced anaphylaxis is a child, to look at the implications for the carer or parent and close family. They may need guidance in how best to care for the child, and support in acknowledging and coping with the psychological stress they may be under. Siblings can also be affected by the frightening consequences of an anaphylactic attack.

The psychological features of anaphylaxis have not been publicised as well as the physical features. However, there is much that can be done to alleviate the fear and restore a person's ability to function normally after an anaphylactic attack. The first, and most important step is for all concerned to recognise and acknowledge the emotional and psychological effects of anaphylaxis.

The Effects on a Person with Anaphylaxis

Generally, people who have experienced an acute anaphylactic attack will have felt close to death. Most people deal remarkably well with this experience. People will initially feel very shaken, but once they have had a chance to consider the situation, and talk things through with their partner, friends, parents or maybe their doctor, they will usually come to terms with their new situation. However, a number of psychological and emotional problems can arise that need particular attention.

ANXIETY

Some people may experience symptoms of anxiety. Some might keep reliving the attack and avoiding reminders of it. Their reaction and the subsequent symptoms could also markedly interfere with their work and social life, and would prevent them carrying out some necessary everyday task. Here are some of the symptoms a person may experience.

- They may keep re-experiencing the attack by continually remembering it, or by having recurrent dreams or flashbacks.
- They may actively avoid anything associated with the attack, including thoughts and feelings that remind them of it, and also activities, places and people.
- They may completely or partially lose their memory of the event.
- They could lose interest in activities that used to be important to them, or feel unable to do them.
- They may feel estranged or detached from people.
- They may express the feeling that they will not live long or

be able to live life fully.
- They may have difficulty falling asleep or staying asleep.
- They may experience irritability or sudden outbursts of anger.
- They may have difficulty concentrating.
- They may be hypervigilant (obsessively aware of everything that is happening around them).
- They may have an exaggerated, startled response to certain things.
- They may react physically (e.g. sweat or hyperventilate) when anything reminds them of the attack.

It is quite possible that they may not experience any of these symptoms following an anaphylactic attack, or only one or two of them. If they have experienced any of these symptoms after an anaphylactic attack, or perhaps they are still experiencing them, it means that they have been very stressed by the experience. This is entirely normal and understandable. It is important to acknowledge the situation so that the issues can be addressed by the loved ones around. Occasionally some people might need professional help.

DENIAL

People who have experienced anaphylaxis may be so successful at driving the experience from their mind that they deny it has happened at all. Alternatively, someone may have have been so stressed by the situation that denial becomes a psychological defence barrier. Whatever the cause this is very dangerous, as shown by Juliet's story below.

JULIET'S STORY

'My first experience of an anaphylactic attack happened in my late twenties. I was stung by a wasp whilst I was out in the garden quite happily enjoying the warm, sunny weather. I felt the sting, followed by an acute burning sensation. I was annoyed for not having seen the wasp as I sipped my drink. Then it hit me. I started to feel dizzy and extremely hot. My skin suddenly became red and blotchy, and I felt my tongue beginning to swell. I felt sick, and then I felt panic. I need help! Luckily my husband was with me and he called our doctor, who, thankfully, lives close by.

'Within a few minutes he arrived and, understanding the seriousness of the situation, gave me an adrenaline injection immediately. Thereafter, I recovered quickly, but it became apparent to me that this was no normal reaction to a wasp sting. I was told that I had had a severe allergic reaction to a wasp sting, in other words, I had an anaphylactic reaction.

'I am now supposed to carry adrenaline injections with me at all times, always wear shoes, keep the windows and doors shut in the summer, and be alert to the danger of wasps. Frankly, I find this very restrictive, and I refuse to allow my life to be ruled by these creatures. I hardly ever carry adrenaline even though my husband reminds me. My view is that if I'm going to be stung that's just too bad. I shall live normally as I have always done, and enjoy myself. Why should I always be on the lookout for danger and make myself a nervous wreck? It's just not practical, and anyway, it is very unlikely that I shall be stung again. I hate injections as well.'

Juliet acknowledges that she has anaphylaxis, but denies how crucial it is to be well prepared for any potential attack. Interestingly, she also admits that she fears injections. This is another factor that anaphylaxis sufferers must deal with. It is probably fair to say that most people dislike injections, and many are actually afraid of them. It is not surprising, there-fore, that some are unwilling to take medication that has been prescribed for them.

Denial enables the person to build a protective facade that allows them to continue with their lives in a relatively normal way. It is important to give such a person support, whilst at the same time helping them to face the reality of their experience. They need to understand that they are putting their lives at risk if they do not take their medication, or if they knowingly expose themselves to the trigger of their anaphylaxis.

Teenagers are particularly susceptible to shutting the door on their anaphylaxis. Educating them as to the best ways of adapting to their condition is crucial. The initial aim must be to restore an acceptable level of safety and control. The carers and loved ones of a family member with anaphylaxis need to be aware of the possible consequences of the sufferer's denial. They must be alert to the danger the person is exposing themselves to, and firmly but sensitively remind them to take their medication, and minimise their exposure to triggers. The advice of carers needs to be adequate, honest, unambiguous, and timely. It is of great importance to provide such a person with a feeling of security and confidence, trust and safety, while helping them to be independent and responsible for their own anaphylaxis.

If the person with anaphylaxis is a child, a great onus is placed on his or her family and carers. They need to be the anaphylactic's eyes and memory, continually alert for them. In the case of a teenager this will sometimes cause friction, even irritation, and great sensitivity is needed. The efforts of carers will help people who have experienced anaphylaxis to face reality and accept their problem, so that they can resume their daily activities as normally as possible.

FEAR

When a person experiences a life-threatening reaction, they may become hypersensitive to anything that reminds them of the event. They may feel fear, terror and extreme anxiety when they encounter these reminders.

One woman who experienced an anaphylactic attack after being stung by a wasp described what happened when she next encountered a wasp:

'My husband had encouraged and finally convinced me to go into town after I had nearly died from a wasp sting. When we arrived at the car park, there it was, flying around the car, just waiting for me to get out. It was coming to get me. I knew it was going to sting me. I could not move. I would not open the door, we had to turn back...'

But it is not only the sufferer who experiences fear. A life-threatening attack has repercussions on the entire family, particularly young children. They are acutely aware of their parents or siblings being frightened or disturbed.

RELATIONSHIP PROBLEMS

Occasionally, after experiencing an anaphylactic attack, some people may have difficulties with their relationships with family, friends and society, and end up feeling very isolated. In some cases, they will retreat into the safety of their immediate family, and their life together, away and protected from the larger community. In other cases, parents may have difficulty in caring for their children, particularly very young ones. People may find relationships at work difficult, and this could even threaten their livelihood.

The Effects on the Carer

The families and carers of children and teenagers who have experienced an anaphylactic attack may be perplexed by the emotional impact, both on themselves, other family members and the child, that may occur following this frightening event. Family members may feel stressed by the whole episode, disrupting the usual pattern of family life. This stress may 'infect' other members of the family. This may cause people to react in unfamiliar ways. This can sometimes express itself in:

- hostility towards each other
- lack of verbal communication
- reduction in expression of physical affection
- unpredictable verbal and physical aggression
- feelings of guilt and responsibility for the traumatic event

The most common problem in the family unit is the mother becoming massively over-protective towards her child. This is perfectly understandable. She sees an already risky world suddenly becoming very dangerous. Her protective instinct can almost smother the child. Perhaps she will not allow the child to stay at friends' houses or go on school trips – indeed she may want to go on the school trips with the child. The mother is trying to establish control over every aspect of the child's life. The father, though less commonly, may become similarly over-protective.

However, a whole range of other problems may occur. For example, if the mother is highly stressed as a result of experiencing an anaphylactic attack herself, or as a result of another member of the family experiencing an anaphylactic attack, a father or older sibling might have to assume the practical and emotional role of a mother. The younger children may get confused and increasingly insecure when their day-to-day routine is suddenly changed. This can result in bed-wetting, physical and verbal withdrawal, disrupted sleep patterns, and refusal to eat or drink. A stressed father often withdraws into the relative security of his job, distancing himself from family members and consequently disrupting the unity of the family.

Children can show signs of stress too. They may feel rejected and, conversely, they may reject other members of their family. This can result in hostility to other family members, poor communication, and fewer expressions of affection.

The stronger the social bonds between friends, family and community, the better the sufferer and their carers will cope with the after-effects of a life-threatening anaphylactic attack. Conversely, if their family and social bonds are weak, and they feel isolated and rejected, they will be more likely to develop emotional and psychological problems.

Emotional and Psychological Support

Clearly anaphylaxis can have a big impact on anyone touched by it. However, by looking honestly at the situation, and discussing any lifestyle changes that are required, both the person who has experienced anaphylaxis and those around him or her, will be able to lead a full and normal life. Expert help is readily at hand. The Anaphylaxis Campaign (see Useful Addresses) has an advice line and up-to-date literature available. Allergy clinics and well-informed GPs are good sources of information.

How anaphylaxis can be successfully integrated into family life with minimal disruption is illustrated by Karen's family.

KAREN'S FAMILY

'Being the parent of a child at risk of food anaphylaxis can be frightening and at times overwhelming. We have two who are allergic to nuts. Perhaps we can share our personal coping strategies.

'David is seven and still very much under our care. We have never prevented him from going to play at his friends' homes or going to parties, school outings or

---

other social occasions. We feel it would be wrong to deprive him of these activities. It is our policy to make sure David understands he is at risk. As a consequence he simply refuses any offers of biscuits or cakes unless he receives assurance from the adult caring for him.

'He never goes anywhere without his Epipen. We borrow the trainer pen from time to time from my husband's surgery and we all, including David, have a practice session. I also visit David's school at least once a term to remind the staff how to use the Epipen and we have given them a clear emergency action plan.

'Dan is 14. He is a keen sportsman and his school sporting commitments often taken him away from home for a few days at a time. The boys are hosted by the families of the home side and yes, we do let him go! Dan's sportsmaster ensures that the host family are fully informed and I always ring them beforehand.

'We know Dan's friends well and have made sure they understand why he carries an Epipen, how and when to use it, and where to find it. As they set off somewhere, I've often heard them asking if he's got his 'pen'.

'By allowing our children such freedom we could be accused of being cavalier. I think not. Life is about calculating the risks and getting on with it. Our children ride bikes, so we make them wear helmets; one of them surfs and we know he can swim; one of them rides horses, she wears a hard hat; two of them are at risk from anaphylaxis, they are vigilant and carry Epipens.'

Strong support from family and friends helps the person affected by anaphylaxis to lead a normal life. It helps them to deal effectively with the legacy of their anaphylactic attack, and enables them to have a positive outlook for the future. A person who has experienced the fear of an anaphylactic attack needs to be encouraged to come to terms with what has happened to them and to help themselves. This will change the person's perspective from that of being controlled by anaphylaxis, to being in control.

However, a few people do need rather more intensive support to help them sort out the emotional and psychological problems that may follow a life-threatening anaphylactic attack. Examples of this type of help include psychotherapy, counselling and behavioural therapy.

PSYCHOTHERAPY

Immediate, problem-orientated, and structured short-term psychotherapy may be of value in dealing with problems associated with an anaphylactic attack. In the UK, this is provided under the NHS and is via a doctor's referral. The individual is encouraged to talk about their experience, to accept their feelings, acknowledge their symptoms and see the effect that anaphylaxis will have on their subsequent life and that of their immediate family or carers. In coming to terms with the impact it has had, they are encouraged to develop an optimistic attitude, to avoid blaming themselves or others, and to accept help and support. Most importantly, they are helped to resume the activities of their daily life as normally as possible.

COUNSELLING

There are different types of counselling available. One-to-one counselling can help the individual initially and increase their confidence. And group therapy can provide some powerful and much-needed support. Group experience lessens the individual's sense of isolation and alienation. Members find that others can understand fear and distress. Social reintegration begins when members feel the support of the group, and come to believe they are no longer facing the problems of recovery by themselves.

BEHAVIOURAL THERAPY

This is an effective treatment for stress, and anxiety disorders particularly generated by any reminder of the anaphylactic attack. Exposure to the situation in which the anaphylactic attack occurred can be an effective treatment, and also exposure to the feared stimuli or trigger, for example, a bee, a wasp or peanuts. Gradual, controlled exposure, under professional guidance, can reduce the negative effect these triggers may have.

An anaphylactic attack can be terrifying, and the emotional and psychological problems it causes can effectively stop the clock for all involved. The primary parental functions of protecting, loving and teaching become disturbed. Both the anaphylactic and their immediate family can be completely disorientated by the experience. Emotional bonds can be greatly strengthened but, conversely, they may be weakened. The family may feel unable to cope with the fluctuating moods of both the anaphylactic, and other family members.

When someone has had such a close brush with death, they may need to seek professional advice and support. They need to see the experience in such a way that they can begin to regard themselves as stronger and wiser and their lives as having a new value. The victim thus gradually becomes the survivor, with an increased feeling of control and a lessening of the fear that the experience will recur.

Dramatic life-threatening events affect families, not just individuals. Treatment should therefore address both the individual and their relationships with others. Group and family therapy can be helpful from this point of view. Learning about stress management, overcoming fear, boosting self-esteem and dealing with the practical disruptions in family life (such as taking special precautions to minimise exposure to triggers) can help the individual and his or her family to deal with the anaphylaxis.

8

ANAPHYLAXIS AND SCHOOLS

A child with anaphylaxis is not 'unwell'. He appears entirely normal, he behaves in a normal way, he is quite able to take part in school activities, just as he could if he were short-sighted or had asthma. His condition is not contagious, he does not need antibiotics, painkillers or other regular medication. Therefore, he should be at school.

Let's assume that your son, Ben, has been diagnosed as severely allergic to peanuts. In all other respects he is a normal, healthy child, but if he eats any peanut product, he will quickly experience a life-threatening allergic reaction.

By now you have probably been well advised by your doctor and allergy specialist, have been taught how to administer adrenaline and are rethinking your family's eating habits so as to avoid peanuts in any shape or form. You have worked hard, and are getting used to living with anaphylaxis. It probably took time, and a fair amount of worry, to come to terms with Ben's anaphylaxis, but you love him and would do anything to ensure his well-being.

If Ben is to lead a normal life, he will have to go to school. But he needs constant, immediate access to adrenaline and, particularly while he is very young, he needs help in avoiding peanuts. In order for Ben to be safe at school, the school will have to play a part in the management of his condition. It would be foolish to assume that, if he does have an anaphylactic reaction, it will only take place when you are around. It is just as likely to happen when he is away from you – perhaps more so – and so other people have to be involved. As a parent, you may need to convince the staff at the school that they can cope with your anaphylactic child.

Because anaphylaxis is not as well-known a condition as, say, asthma, it is quite likely that your first hurdle will be that of communication. You are asking Ben's teachers to understand all about anaphylaxis, a condition they may never even have heard of, and then to shoulder the problem. It is not surprising that they may, initially, be unwilling to get involved. This is where good communication is so vital.

Meeting the Head Teacher

The first step is to arrange a meeting with the head teacher. He may well ask Ben's form teacher, the school nurse or perhaps the deputy head to attend. It would be helpful if Ben's doctor could also attend, although this may not be practical. Your task is to convince the head that, far from being a rare or unknown condition, anaphylaxis is well-documented and on the increase. It may be worth making the following points:

- It is thought that around 30,000 people in Britain suffer extreme allergic reactions to nuts.
- Many deaths that were once attributed to asthma are now thought to have resulted from anaphylactic shock.
- There are other factors which can also provoke an anaphylactic attack, such as other foodstuffs, bee and wasp stings and latex.
- An emergency may never arise. But if it does, a sensible management plan would reduce risks to a minimum.

Also, the authorities are keen to ensure that schools are informed about anaphylaxis. In Britain, the Department for Education and Employment and the Department of Health have included anaphylaxis in a document entitled *Supporting Children with Medical Needs in School*. If your school does not have this guide, it can be obtained from the Department for Education and Employment (see Useful Addresses).

This guide states that: 'Children with special medical needs have the same rights of admission to school as other children, and cannot generally be excluded from school for medical reasons.' At the same time, it says that: 'There is no legal duty which requires school staff to administer medication; this is a voluntary role.' In other words, your child is going to need the teachers to be prepared to administer adrenaline should an emergency arise, and the teachers are not legally obliged to do this. This is where you, or perhaps a healthcare professional, need to reassure them that they can be trained to carry out this simple procedure.

Above all, your meeting should not be a confrontational, 'I know-my-rights' type of encounter, but an attempt to form an alliance with the school that will be in Ben's best interests. It is worth remembering that, if the school does not have an anaphylaxis policy, it is probably because it has not previously had a pupil with anaphylaxis, rather than because it is reluctant to tackle the issue.

Apart from the Education Department guidelines some local education authorities also produce guidelines for schools in their area. When you meet the head teacher, you may be pleasantly surprised to find that his local authority has already given him guidance.

WHO MAKES THE POLICIES?

In Britain, state schools and local authorities form their own policies, reflecting legal obligations and their own particular situations. They are responsible for the health

---

and safety of pupils in their care. The Health and Safety at Work Act (1974) makes employers responsible for the health and safety of their employees and anyone else on the premises. In schools this covers the head and teachers, non-teaching staff, pupils and visitors. Who 'the employer' is depends on the type of school:

- The local education authority is the employer in county and controlled schools.
- The governing body is the employer in City Technology Colleges, voluntary aided and grant maintained schools.
- The proprietor or the trustees are the employers in some independent schools.

At the meeting, the following questions may be raised:

- Does Ben need medicine every day? *No.*
- Can other pupils catch anaphylaxis? *No.*
- In an emergency, are you expecting a member of staff to give an injection? *Yes, but not the sort of injection you are probably used to. Not haphazardly jabbing a child with a needle and plunging in a syringe. We can arrange training, and will suppy pre-loaded devices containing the correct doses of adrenaline. In an emergency, you simple remove the cap and push the device, through clothing if need be, against the child's thigh. The rest happens automatically.*
- Are you expecting the school to keep information about Ben's condition confidential? *No. People in a position of responsibility for Ben need to be aware. We could arrange a talk by our doctor or allergy nurse so that all involved understand how even the merest trace of peanut could be dangerous to Ben.*

Drawing Up a Plan

Having established that anaphylaxis is a known medical condition which can be accommodated within the school, and that the school is willing to learn about and deal with Ben's situation, you need to draw up a plan. Here the Education Department guidelines will be useful, as they contain sample healthcare plans and forms which can be adapted to fit Ben's needs.

The agreed document should include accurate details of Ben's condition, medication, contact phone numbers and addresses for his doctor and parents. There should be a request for the school to administer medication, staff training records and confirmation of the head teacher's agreement to administer medication. The school may well have an Emergency Planning protocol for calling an ambulance, explaining where the school entrance is, describing symptoms, and other vital information. If it does not, this information should also be included in Ben's plan.

Once the basic plan has been drawn up, you can work out the details of excluding and avoiding peanuts. As we saw in Chapter 6, it is relatively simple to monitor a child's diet if they are only eating freshly prepared foods. However, hidden dangers abound as soon as they encounter packaged, pre-cooked food. It is the same at school. Added peanuts can be eliminated from school meals, but has the cook remembered the hidden dangers such as the oil which has previously been used for cooking nut products?

There will be occasions when Ben might encounter peanuts, perhaps in another pupil's packed lunch, or on a school outing. Here awareness and vigilance among staff, parents and other pupils is vital. Everyone who is responsible for Ben during a school day – and afterwards if he is going somewhere other than home – needs to be informed about his anaphylaxis, and how even the merest trace of peanut might affect him.

IS THE TEACHER LIABLE IF SOMETHING GOES WRONG?

Even if a school is anaphylaxis-aware, even if the caterers avoid allergens and the staff are trained in administering adrenaline, mistakes can be made. There is always the remote possibility that, for some reason, the school could fail to help a child suffering anaphylactic shock. Teachers can be reassured that, usually, their employer will insure against this happening and will assume responsibility in any subsequent legal action. This protection is called *indemnity*. The head teacher should always check that his staff are covered in this way before they agree to administer adrenaline.

PERSONALISING THE PLAN

If Ben's school has responded in the way you hoped, the head will agree a protocol and one or two willing teachers will be trained to administer Ben's adrenaline. Remember that the plan of action for Ben will differ from that for another child with similar problems.

For example, we have repeatedly said in this book that people who need adrenaline injections must always carry them on their person. But is Ben old enough to cope with this responsibility? Even if you feel he is, what about his classmates? Might one of them succumb to curiosity, and secretly tamper with the medication? If this could occur, it might be safer if there were several doses of adrenaline, each held by different teachers or at different locations.

Also, consider what happens if the school needs to contact you in an emergency. Are you always available? Does the school have any alternative people to contact if they cannot find you? Does Ben know about these other people, and how would he feel if they travelled to hospital with him instead of you? A solution might be for you to always carry a mobile phone, although this is expensive and not infallible. It is simply important to remember that you have entered into a partnership with the school, and must play your part as actively and responsibly as members of the school play theirs.

Who Else Needs to Know About Anaphylaxis?

It is not only parents of children with anaphylaxis, or schools with anaphylactic pupils, who need to be aware of this condition. A child may experience her first ever anaphylactic reaction at school. In this case there might not be an agreed protocol, handy adrenaline, or a trained administrator. In this event, it would be vital to follow the emergency procedures described in Chapter 5.

Anaphylaxis does not just happen in schools. There are many situations where children are supervised by adults other than their parents. These could include playgroups, crèches, nurseries, Brownie pack holidays, Scout camps, activity weekends, Sunday schools – even birthday parties. Your nanny, au pair or babysitter assumes responsibility for your child if you are not there. Do they know what to do in an emergency? Do they know that there could be peanuts in supermarket bread, or chocloate bars?

You need to inform all those around your anaphylactic child about his condition, how to avoid it and how to treat it. Similarly, *anyone* who takes responsibility for other peoples' children would benefit from knowing about anaphylaxis and how to cope with it.

IN CONCLUSION

Anaphylaxis is far more common than people think. Indeed, the widespread and increasing incidence of anaphylaxis may well turn out to be helpful to those who have been coping with it for a long time already. The more people know about anaphylaxis, the more likely they are to know how to avoid it or what to do in an emergency. But the increase in anaphylaxis is also likely to lead to a further stretching of health service resources, as the demand for allergy clinics, medication and specialist help increases.

The louder the collective 'voice' of people with anaphylaxis, the more likely it is to have an impact. For example, at present, food retailers discourage people with anaphylaxis from buying certain goods by warning them that they might contain traces of allergen. There must be a point of demand at which it becomes economically preferable for food producers to take the next step and use dedicated production lines to ensure that food is free from allergens, thus encouraging these customers.

Food producers and retailers must not be allowed to forget about anaphylaxis. The controversial moves towards allowing genetic modification of food has wide implications for people with anaphylaxis. It has already been shown that when a protein from brazil nuts was introduced into soya beans, people who were allergic to brazil nuts became allergic to the soya. Without adequate labelling, there is no way of telling whether or not the food you are eating has been genetically modified.

As the worldwide consumption of peanuts rises, so does the incidence of peanut-induced anaphylaxis. With increased information about anaphylaxis, mothers would know not to eat peanuts during pregnancy and breastfeeding, and not to give peanut butter to young babies. Again, awareness is vital.

The search for new ways of dealing with anaphylaxis continues. Ideas under the spotlight include an anti-allergy vaccine that could destroy the allergy antibodies, a user-friendly kit for discovering the tiniest traces of particular allergens in food, and easier ways of giving adrenaline. These and other innovations may one day help to protect us from the condition of *excessive protection* – anaphylaxis.

GLOSSARY

ADRENALINE: A hormone produced by the body in response to stress.

ALLERGEN: The factor which provokes an inappropriate inflammatory response.

ALLERGIC: If a factor provokes an inappropriate inflammatory response, you are said to be allergic to that factor.

ALVEOLI: Air-filled sacs at the end of the bronchioles.

ANAPHYLAXIS: A condition which causes severe, systemic, life-threatening allergic reactions.

ASTHMA: A disease in which inflammation of the airways causes breathing difficulties, wheezing and constriction of the chest.

ATOPIC TENDENCY: If a person's body contains genes which predispose them to develop allergies, they are said to have an atopic tendency.

BRONCHI: The two main branches of the trachea.

BRONCHIOLES: Small sub-divisions of the bronchial tubes.

DENIAL: A pattern of behaviour in which people refuse to admit the reality or existence of something. Some people with anaphylaxis deny that they have a problem, and refuse to carry the medication that might save their lives if they had a bad attack.

ECZEMA: Inflammation of the skin, causing redness, swelling and cracking.

EXTRACTABLE PROTEINS: Natural impurities in latex which are known triggers of anaphylaxis.

FOOD ADDITIVES: Substances used to preserve or enhance food. Some additives are known to trigger anaphylaxis.

INFLAMMATORY MEDIATORS: Powerful chemicals which circulate in the blood stream, passing through blood vessel walls and between cells. They are an integral part of the inflammatory response.

INFLAMMATORY RESPONSE: The response our bodies use to protect us from hostile factors in the environment.

LATEX: The whitish, milky fluid that is produced by many plants. It is the latex from the rubber tree *hevea braziliensis* that can cause anaphylaxis.

LUMEN: The hollow part of the airways.

METERED DOSE INHALER (MDI): A type of inhaler used in anaphylaxis to deliver adrenaline to the surface of the lungs. An MDI is a metal canister encased in a plastic shell. The medication is released in the form of an aerosol spray.

PSYCHOLOGY: The study of human and animal behaviour. Psychological factors such as stress and depression are linked to anaphylaxis.

SYSTEMIC: A reaction that occurs throughout the entire body.

TRACHEA: The tube which takes air from the larynx to the bronchi. Its non-technical name is windpipe.

WEALS: Water blisters in the skin, sometimes called hives or nettle rash.

USEFUL ADDRESSES

The Anaphylaxis Campaign
PO Box 149
Fleet
Hampshire GU13 9XU
Tel: 01252 318723

The British Allergy Foundation
23 Middle Street
London EC1A 7JA
Tel: 0171-600 6166

British Red Cross Contact your local Branch Head-quarters, listed in the telephone directory

British Society for Allergy and Clinical Immunology
(*for handbook of clinicians and scientists in the UK and overseas*)
66 Weston Park
Thames Ditton
Surrey KT7 0HL
Tel: 0181-398 9240

Department for Education and Employment
(*for document 'Supporting Children with Medical Needs in Schools'*)

Sanctuary Buildings
Great Smith Street
London SW1P 3BT
Tel: 0171-925 5555

Two Ten
Department of Health
(*For copies of 'Latex Sensitisation in the Health Care Setting'.*
This is free of charge to the National Health Service if a
written request, quoting reference MDA DB 9601, is sent.)
PO Box 410
Wetherby
Yorkshire LS23 7EL

Otherwise, copies can be obtained for £10.00 from:
The Medical Devices Agency
Ordering Department, Room 1207
Hannibal House
Elephant and Castle
London SE1 6TQ
Tel: 0171-972 8181

Derma Prene synthetic polymer gloves can be bought
from Surgicon Ltd. Tel: 01484 712147

The Food Intolerance Databank
Scientific and Technical Information
Leatherhead Food RA
Randalls Road
Leatherhead
Surrey KT22 7RY
Tel: 01372 376761

MedicAlert Foundation
1 Bridge Wharf
156 Caledonian Road
London N1 9UU
Tel: 0171-833 3034

For the leaflet on food additives (in England and Wales)
Ministry of Agriculture, Fisheries and Food
Publications Unit
Lion House
Willowburn Trading Estate
Alnwick
Northumberland NE66 2PF

(in Scotland)
Scottish Home and Health Department
Foods Branch
Room 44
St Andrew's House
Edinburgh EH1 3DE

(in Northern Ireland)
The Department of Health and Social Services
Food Control Branch
Annex A
Dundonald House
Upper Newtownards Road
Belfast BT4 3SF

The National Asthma Campaign
Providence House
Providence Place
London N1 0NT
Tel: 0171-226 2260

St Andrew's Ambulance Association Your local
Committee Secretary will be listed in the telephone directory

St John Ambulance Your local division will be listed in the
telephone directory

INDEX

INDEX